Preventing
Nursing with Infectious Patients

Kim Maryniak • Robbie Garrett

Preventing Errors and Pitfalls in Nursing with Infectious Patients

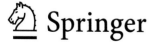 Springer

Kim Maryniak
Independent Consultants
Casa Grande, AZ, USA

Robbie Garrett
Independent Consultants
Casa Grande, AZ, USA

ISBN 978-3-030-86727-0   ISBN 978-3-030-86728-7   (eBook)
https://doi.org/10.1007/978-3-030-86728-7

This Springer imprint is published by the registered company Springer Nature
Switzerland AG
The registered company address is: Gewerbestrasse 11, 6330 Cham, Switzerland

Special thanks to our peer reviewers:
Charene Dehne, BSN, RN,
EMT-Paramedic, Lt.
Kiersten Fink, BSN, RN

Preface

Nurses play the largest role in patient care and nursing continues to be the most trusted profession. With current staffing shortages worldwide, patients who are sicker and with higher acuity, and more task-oriented duties assigned to nurses, the capacity to balance everything can be tedious. The overwhelming workload may sometimes contribute to errors, ranging from minor to irreversible, or even fatal consequences. There is a great deal of responsibility on nurses to avoid errors. The aim of *Preventing Errors and Pitfalls in Nursing with Infectious Patients* is to inform nurses about the most common and the more serious errors made in caring for patients with infectious diseases, and strategies to help reduce these errors.

The use of just culture will be discussed, and how that framework can be used to determine cause of errors and the potential need for system and process improvements. Factors that are predisposing and contributing factors for nursing errors will be reviewed. This can include personal factors, such as health or knowledge, processes, and environmental factors. Or a combination of factors can exist, which can create a higher risk for errors.

This book covers learnings about a variety of infectious diseases, including COVID-19, multidrug-resistant organisms (MDROs) such as methicillin-resistant Staphylococcus aureus (MRSA), vancomycin-resistant Enterococcus (VRE), Clostridium difficile (C-diff.), and tuberculosis (TB), among others. Infectious diseases will be discussed in terms of causes, symptoms, management, and isolation requirements.

The types of errors, consequences, detection, and monitoring for nursing errors will be included. There are multiple types of errors that can occur during the care of infectious patients, which may be in relation to precautions and isolation processes. Other errors may also occur, such as those attributing to hospital-acquired conditions, falls, or medication errors. There can be multiple consequences as a result of nursing errors, which can affect the patient, family, and even the healthcare professionals involved. Negative affects at an organization-wide level may also occur as a result of errors. There are a variety of strategies that can be implemented to detect and monitor for nursing errors. Process improvement and quality assurance through use of effective tools can assist with detection and monitoring of errors. System tactics and effective communication are also vital to make improvements. A workplace culture that is supportive with effective leadership can also assist in reduction of errors.

The book will describe how errors can be avoided with necessary precautions and managed appropriately based on current evidence-based practice. There are many practices that have been identified in studies to help prevent nursing errors. Some examples of strategies include reduction of hospital-acquired conditions, falls, or other forms of patient harm through the use of bundles. System and personal considerations can also prevent nursing errors.

Case studies and examples will be provided, demonstrating effective practices for reducing patient errors with infectious patients. Recommendations for further study are also provided.

Casa Grande, AZ, USA   Kim Maryniak
                                                        Robbie Garrett

Contents

Contributing Factors for Nursing Errors

1

There are multiple factors that influence whether or not nursing errors occur. It is important to view errors in terms of a "just culture," where the focus should be on improving patient safety rather than blame. Just culture looks at accountability and faults within systems; fingers are not pointed to blame one individual. Often processes need improving, or education is lacking. However, it is not a blame-free environment; if there is an individual's responsibility, then that person must have accountability (Marx 2001; Maryniak 2019).

Within the just culture framework, incidents are reviewed based on duties, rather than the outcome. Duties of an individual include a duty to produce an outcome, a duty to follow a procedural rule, and a duty to avoid unjustifiable risk. For a duty to produce an outcome, there are no specific procedures or steps in how to do something, but as an individual, it is expected that you will have a defined result. There may be an acceptable rate of failure for expectations. With a duty to follow a procedural rule, the expectation is that as an individual, we are expected to follow a procedure or policy in a specific way. And the duty to avoid unjustifiable risk is described as an overarching duty for everyone. As individuals, generally, we do not do anything that is intentionally reckless, but there are times when we may need to make

K. Maryniak, R. Garrett, *Preventing Errors and Pitfalls in Nursing with Infectious Patients*, https://doi.org/10.1007/978-3-030-86728-7_1

a choice to do the right thing, but may breach and harm another value in the process; this is considered justifiable (Marx 2001; Maryniak 2019; Paradiso and Sweeney 2019; Rogers et al. 2017).

There are reasons why a breach of duty may occur, which include human error, at-risk behavior, and reckless behavior. Human error is known as an inadvertent action, or a slip, lapse or mistake. In these circumstances, a genuine mistake is made. This may include a skill-based mistake, an omission or forgetfulness, or a knowledge-based error. An example of a human error is a nurse who is drawing up a medication in the medication room and is interrupted. When she asks her coworker to verify the dose, it is pointed out that she has drawn up the incorrect amount.

At-risk behavior is described as when someone chooses to do something that can inadvertently increase the chance for harm to occur. The potential for harm is added but is not recognized by the person who is drifting away from consciously safer choices. The individual is aware that behavior is drifting away from set practices, such as creating a workaround for a process. Many times, at-risk behaviors begin with system problems, such as ineffective processes, delays, or equipment problems. A workaround is found to deal with the system issue, but it creates behavior that becomes dangerous. One example is that there are not enough barcode scanners on a particular unit. As a workaround, to ensure medications are given on time, nurses begin to override the barcode scanning, rather than waiting to use the scanner. This is a system problem (not enough barcode scanners), but the nurses have found a workaround that is at-risk behavior.

With reckless behavior, an individual actually chooses an action that knowingly puts themselves or others in harm's way. The risk is identified but ignored. The individual is aware that their behavior is reckless, and there is a conscious disregard of others. One example is narcotic diversion. The nurse is aware that it is illegal but does not stop the behavior.

Repetitive errors with patient safety also need to be addressed. Even if it is a human error each time, repetitiveness indicates a deeper problem. An example is a nurse who has repeated medication errors. The root is determined to be human error each time, and yet there are still multiple occasions of the issue, which increases the patient risk (Marx 2001; Maryniak 2019; Paradiso and Sweeney 2019; Rogers et al. 2017).

When looking at how nursing errors occur, it is important to understand which contributing factors are involved. Contributing factors are those that can cause an error or determine the level of risk, directly or indirectly. An error may be a result of one or a combination of contributing factors, which may be related to human, environmental, or organizational considerations.

Human errors such as slips and lapses were identified in studies as a common cause of nursing errors. Human errors are more seen with personal and environmental factors as contributing causes. Health status of staff is a condition that can lead to slips and lapses. This included tiredness, fatigue, sleep deprivation, and illness.

Physical signs, including indications of burnout, noted in studies may or may not be related to long hours and lack of breaks. Stress at work, lack of assertiveness, and personality also contributed to personal health. A busy work environment, distractions, interruptions, and pressure from others or time limitations can also increase the likelihood of human errors. Skill mix and workload are commonly identified as contributing to errors. This includes the volume of admissions, discharges, and transfer. Staffing with heavy patient loads and multitasking were other factors. Omissions and violations occurred more often. Patient acuity was another condition identified as a contributing factor. This was particularly true when combined with other factors, particularly with wrong time or dose omission. Short staffing was also a factor, particularly when added to skill mix of staff, workload, and patient acuity (Donaldson et al. 2021; Roth et al. 2017).

Examples of slips and lapses involving medications include misidentifying either medication or patient. Contributing causes were misreading labels or documentation, look-a-like sound-a-like medications or patient names, lack of concentration, complacency, and carelessness. In terms of errors associated with infectious diseases, slip and errors can contribute to inappropriate donning and doffing, for example. Further descriptions of errors will be covered in Chap. 3.

Knowledge-based mistakes were also noted in studies, but less frequent. This included lack of knowledge about isolation requirements, understanding about medications being administered or equipment that was being used, as well as unfamiliarity with patient. Lack of critical thinking may be related to knowledge, personal, or environmental factors (Donaldson et al. 2021; Roth et al. 2017).

Written communication in studies included illegible and unclear documentation. Transcription errors also contributed to medication and procedure errors. These types of contributing factors were associated with facilities that still use written documentation, or during downtime procedures. Other sources of inadequate written communication were a lack of appropriate policies, procedures, or protocols. Verbal communication, such as handoffs or interdisciplinary communications, was also noted in studies as contributions to errors (Krein et al. 2018; Roth et al. 2017).

Supplies and storage are also associated with errors. Logistics related to a unit or ward stock contributed to errors with medication and procedure times or omission, including medication or supply misplacement. Delays in delivery of medication or treatment, or unavailable medications and supplies were also sources of errors. Difficulties with equipment is another contributing condition to errors. Malfunctioning equipment, unfamiliarity or unclear equipment design, and insufficient availability of equipment contributed to errors (Donaldson et al. 2021; Krein et al. 2018).

Deliberate violations were not commonly seen in studies, and do not infer that there was malicious or ill intent. Violations were occurrences in which the nurses knew that processes were not followed. Violations of processes were situational and were related to trusting colleagues, lack of appropriate protocols, patient acuity, and staff. The violations noted in studies related to medication errors were intentionally giving medications early or late, and administering medication without a signed order. Errors related to infectious diseases can include not wearing the appropriate personal protective equipment (PPE) or lack of hand hygiene (Krein et al. 2018).

Reckless behaviors that lead to errors can include the use of controlled substances at work, deliberately tampering with equipment or medications, or knowingly practicing outside of the scope of practice. These types of behaviors are not typical but are dealt with punitively (Rogers et al. 2017).

References

Donaldson L., Ricciardi W., Sheridan, S., & Tartaglia, R. (eds). (2021). *Textbook of patient safety and clinical risk management*. Springer.

Krein, S. L., Mayer, J., Harrod, M., Weston, L. E., Gregory, L., Petersen, L., Samore, M. H., & Drews, F. A. (2018). Identification and characterization of failures in infectious agent transmission precaution practices in hospitals: A qualitative study. *JAMA Internal Medicine*, *178*(8), 1016–1057.

Marx, D. (2001). *Patient safety and the just culture: A primer for health care executives*. Trustees of Columbia University.

Maryniak, K. (2019). *Professional nursing practice in the United States: An overview for international nurses, and those along the continuum from new graduates to experienced nurses*. Author.

Paradiso, L., & Sweeney, N. (2019). Just culture. *Nursing Management 50*(6), 38-45.

Rogers, E., Griffin, E., Carnie, W., Melucci, J., & Weber, R. J. (2017). A Just culture approach to managing medication errors. *Hospital Pharmacy*, *52*(4), 308–315.

Roth, C., Brewer, M., & Wieck, K. L. (2017). Using a Delphi method to identify human factors contributing to nursing errors. *Nursing Forum*, *52*(3), 173–179.

Overview of Specific Infectious Diseases

2

COVID 19

Coronaviruses are a family of viruses that have multiple strains. Forms of coronavirus include severe acute respiratory syndrome (SARS) and Middle East respiratory syndrome (MERS). COVID 19 is a result of the SARS-CoV-2 strain. COVID 19 was first identified in 2019 and quickly became a worldwide pandemic. COVID 19 is spread by droplets or through contaminated surfaces (Centers for Disease Control and Prevention [CDC] 2021a).

Management of COVID 19 with hospitalized patients depends on the severity of the illness. Patients who do not require oxygen may or may not be treated with remdesivir, related to their risk for disease progression. Corticosteroids, including dexamethasone, are not recommended for those patients not requiring oxygen. Recommendations for patients in acute care who do require oxygen include the use of dexamethasone, remdesivir, or a combination thereof. Patients who require high flow oxygen or other noninvasive oxygen delivery, such as bilevel positive airway pressure (BiPAP), should also receive dexamethasone and/or remdesivir. Additionally, these patients should have either baricitinib or tocilizumab given with treatment. Hospitalized patients requiring mechanical ventilation or extracorporeal membrane oxygenation

(ECMO) require dexamethasone and tocilizumab or sarilumab (National Institutes of Health 2021).

Hospitalized patients with COVID 19 also require the management of comorbidities, such as cardiovascular disease, diabetes, chronic obstructive pulmonary disease (COPD), and renal disease. Severe COVID 19 illness can affect multiple organ systems. Patients need to be assessed for additional respiratory disorders such as respiratory distress, sepsis and septic shock, cardiac dysfunction, and diseases of the renal, hepatic, and central nervous systems. Management of each of these issues is imperative (National Institutes of Health 2021).

COVID 19 patients in acute care, particularly intensive care, also have a higher risk of developing hospital-acquired infections such as hospital-acquired pneumonia and ventilator-associated pneumonia. Empiric broad-spectrum antibiotics may be warranted, with a focus on antibiotic stewardship to avoid complications. Hospitalized patients should also have strategies in place to prevent venous thromboembolism (VTE) (National Institutes of Health 2021).

Management of pain and sedation is also essential for hospitalized COVID 19 patients. Spontaneous awakening and breathing trials and early mobility strategies are important considerations. Involvement of family and empowering them in decision-making is significant (National Institutes of Health 2021).

Isolation for COVID 19 patients who do not have aerosol-generating procedures (AGPs) and are not ventilated should be placed in contact plus droplet precautions. Healthcare professionals working with these patients should use personal protective equipment (PPE) including gloves, gowns, and eye protection (such as safety goggles or face shield); N95 masks are recommended, but the use of surgical masks are found to be just as effective according to current studies (National Institutes of Health 2021).

For patients who have AGPs done, the use of airborne precautions is recommended, including placement of patients in negative-pressure rooms. AGPs include intubation, extubation, induction of sputum, airway suctioning, manual ventilation, continuous positive airway pressure (CPAP), BiPAP, bronchoscopy, and cardiopulmonary resuscitation. It is recommended that AGPs be limited to COVID 19 patients. Healthcare professionals should wear PPE for contact precautions, and must wear either N95 masks or powered air-purifying respirators (PAPRs). Workers must be fit tested to determine the appropriate N95 mask to wear (National Institutes of Health 2021).

Multidrug-resistant Organisms (MDROs)

Multidrug-resistant organisms (MDROs) are those organisms that are resistant to more than one class of antimicrobial medications. The organisms, usually bacteria, can be easily transmitted between individuals. Hospitalized patients have lower resistance and higher risk for exposure to MDROs, which can also increase the severity of infections (CDC 2019).

Methicillin-resistant Staphylococcus aureus (MRSA) is a bacterial infection that is resistant to beta-lactam antibiotics, including those in the penicillin family such as methicillin. Other versions of Staphylococcus aureus infections may have an intermediate (VISA) or resistance to vancomycin (VRSA) as well. Vancomycin resistant enterococcus (VRE) is another type of MDRO, with the pathogen being resistant to vancomycin (CDC 2019).

Antibiotic stewardship, including cautious and appropriate use of antibiotics, is essential to help prevent development of MDROs. Monitoring antibiotic usage and discontinuing as soon as able are essential strategies. Education of providers and nurses are important considerations. Additionally, organizational factors such as staffing, intra-facility, and interfacility communications about infectious status, and adherence to infection control measures are vital to preventing transmission of MDROs (CDC 2019).

Patients diagnosed with an MDRO require contact isolation, in an attempt to prevent transmission of the organism either through direct or indirect contact with contamination. Gowns and gloves are required for healthcare professionals working with MDRO patients and in an isolation environment. Placement of patients in a single room is preferred, although cohorting may be an option in

consultation with the infection control department. Contact precautions are recommended for patients with MDRO infection and
colonization. Masks and eye protection are warranted if there may
be exposure to droplets, such as during suctioning or other similar
procedures (CDC 2017).

Staphylococcal Disease

Staphylococcus aureus (S. aureus) is the most pathogenic of the
group of staphylococci, which are gram-positive aerobic organisms. Staphylococci are commonly colonized in healthy adults,
particularly the nares and on the skin. Higher carrier rates in hospitalized patients or healthcare professionals can lead to the transmission of *S. aureus* and create hospital-acquired infections. The
populations which are at high risk for *S. aureus* infections include
neonates, breastfeeding mothers, patients with chronic respiratory
disorders, individuals with diabetes mellitus, patients with cancer,
those who have had a transplant, patients with implants or central
lines, postsurgical patients, immunocompromised patients,
patients taking steroids, individuals who are intravenous drug
users, dialysis patients, and patients with wounds or burns. These
vulnerable patients can easily develop a hospital-acquired infection from *S. aureus*, with the transmission most commonly from a
healthcare professional (Bush and Vazquez-Pertejo 2021; Taylor
and Unakal 2021).

Staphylococcal disease occurs through either direct tissue
invasion or exotoxin production of S. aureus. If acquired through
direct tissue invasion, which is most common, then the patient can
develop infections of the skin, pneumonia, endocarditis, osteomyelitis, or septic arthritis. Exotoxin production occasionally occurs,
which can create systemic effects, including toxic shock syndrome, scalded skin syndrome, or food poisoning (Bush and
Vazquez-Pertejo 2021; Taylor and Unakal 2021).

Management of staphylococcal disease involves providing
antibiotics. Although staphylococcal disease is not the same as
methicillin-resistant Staphylococcus aureus (MRSA), it is
assumed that S. aureus infections will be resistant to penicillin G,

amoxicillin, ampicillin, and antipseudomonal penicillins. Antibiotic choices for S. aureus may include penicillinase-resistant penicillins, cephalosporins, carbapenems, tetracyclines, macrolides, fluoroquinolones, trimethoprim/sulfamethoxazole, gentamicin, vancomycin, and teicoplanin. The antibiotic choice is made generally on the basis of infection site, severity, and probability of resistance. See also section on Multidrug-resistant organisms (MDROs). Additional management strategies are based on the site and severity of the infection. Skin debridement, abscess drainage, and wound care may be required. If an intravascular catheter is involved, such as a central line, then it must be removed (Bush and Vazquez-Pertejo 2021; Taylor and Unakal 2021).

Isolation depends on the site and severity of the infection. The CDC recommendations for isolation (2019) are delineated based on these factors. If S. aureus infections are not described in the following list, then only standard precautions are required. For S. aureus with major skin, wound, or burn, contact plus standard precautions are required for the duration of the illness, or until drainage stops or can be contained by the use of a dressing. For staphylococcal disease with minor or limited skin, wound, or burn infection, only standard precautions are needed if a dressing covers and contains any drainage adequately. With scalded skin syndrome, contact plus standard precautions are to be used for the duration of the infection. If there is an outbreak of scalded skin syndrome in a nursery or neonatal intensive care unit (NICU), healthcare professionals should be considered as the potential source. Enterocolitis from staphylococcal disease requires standard precautions, and contact precautions if the patient is diapered or incontinent for the duration of the illness (CDC 2019).

Staphylococcal furunculosis

Staphylococcal furunculosis is development of furuncles, which are also known as boils, most commonly found on the body with hair, friction, and moisture. These painful swellings form an abscess in a hair follicle, with staphylococcus aureus as the cause. The infection can affect the whole hair follicle and subcutaneous tissue. Several furuncles together in adjoining hair follicles which create a deep mass with multiple points of drainage is known as a carbuncle. Furunculosis can also cause cellulitis. Comorbidities such as diabetes, HIV, or intravenous drug use may exist. Antibiotic treatment is required for management; pus drained from the wound(s) may be cultured (Papadakis et al. 2020).

With adult patients, standard precautions are used, although contact may be warranted if drainage is not controlled. Staphylococcal furunculosis in infants and young children requires contact plus standard isolation for the duration of the illness until the wounds stop draining (CDC 2019).

Streptococcal Disease (Group A)

Group A streptococcal infections are caused by the streptococcus pyogenes bacterium. Streptococci is a common pathogen that can cause a variety of infections, most commonly acute pharyngitis. Other infections associated with group A streptococcus include impetigo, cellulitis, necrotizing fasciitis, streptococcal bacteremia, pneumonia, osteomyelitis, otitis media, sinusitis, and meningitis. Long-term effects may include acute glomerulonephritis, acute renal failure, toxic shock syndrome, and rheumatic heart disease (Khan 2021).

Management of group A streptococcus infections depends on the location and severity of the infection. Aspiration of the skin or abscess is often required, and in some cases surgical drainage or debridement is needed. A lumbar puncture, thoracentesis, intubation, fasciotomy, or amputation may also be required (Khan 2021).

Isolation and precautions are also based on the course of the infection. For a major skin, wound, or burn group A streptococcus infection, contact, droplet, and standard precautions are required until 24 h after initiation of effective therapy, or until the drainage stops or can be contained by a dressing. For a minor skin wound or burn only standard precautions are needed if a dressing covers and contains drainage (CDC 2019).

Endometritis or puerperal sepsis from group A streptococcus requires standard precautions only. Pharyngitis or scarlet fever in infants and young children needs droplet plus standard precautions until 24 h after initiation of effective therapy. Pneumonia or serious invasive disease from group A streptococcus also requires droplet plus standard precautions until 24 h of effective therapy. It is noted that outbreaks of serious invasive disease have occurred secondary to transmission among patients and healthcare professionals (CDC 2019).

Clostridium difficile (C-diff)

Clostridium difficile (C-diff.) is an anaerobic bacterium that is gram-positive and forms spores, which causes diarrhea associated with antibiotics and pseudomembranous colitis. C-diff causes a high risk of an outbreak in healthcare settings such as acute care facilities. The risks for developing C. diff increase with multiple courses or prolonged use of broad-spectrum antibiotics. The antibiotics most associated with C. diff are vancomycin, clindamycin, fluoroquinolones, and third-generation cephalosporins (CDC 2019).

Management of C. diff includes stopping the original causative antibiotics if able. Treatment with vancomycin or fidaxomicin is recommended. Bezlotuxumab has also been approved for C. diff management along with the suggested antibiotics. Anti-diarrheal medications should not be used in patients with C. diff. A fecal microbiota transplant (FMT) may also be used by administering healthy stool into the colon of a patient with a C. diff infection (Grinspan 2021).

Contact precautions and isolation are required for patients with C. diff infections, preferably in a single room. There are additional considerations with contact isolation and C. diff patients, formerly known as enteric precautions. Hand hygiene must be performed with handwashing, as alcohol gel may not eliminate the C. diff spores. Disposable equipment should be used with C. diff isolation. Cleaning and sterilization practices need a bleach-based solution, as the spores are also resistant to many other standard solutions (CDC 2019).

Noroviruses

Noroviruses are a set of single-strand RNA viruses that cause acute gastroenteritis. The virus causes symptoms of watery diarrhea, cramping, low-grade fever, and myalgia for up to 60–72 h. Norovirus is highly contagious through direct contact or through droplets spread with vomiting (Khan 2018).

Management of norovirus includes replacement of fluids and electrolytes. In some cases, intravenous fluids are required. Antiemetics for nausea and vomiting and analgesics for myalgia can also be administered (Khan 2018).

Contact isolation is required for hospitalized patients with a norovirus. Patients should be in a single room with a dedicated toilet and equipment. Healthcare professionals should use PPE for contact isolation. Masks are recommended if around a patient with active vomiting. Masks are also recommended for cleaning rooms of a patient with norovirus due to potential droplet spread from body fluids. Contact precautions should be continued for at least 48 h after symptoms have resolved (CDC 2019; Khan 2018).

Rotavirus

Rotavirus, a double-stranded RNA, is another type of virus which causes gastroenteritis. Diarrhea is the primary symptom, which can be profuse, and often leads to dehydration. Nausea, vomiting, low-grade fever, anorexia, and cramping are also seen (Nguyen 2018).

Management of rotavirus includes replacement of fluids and electrolytes, and intravenous fluids are frequently required to prevent dehydration. Antiemetics for nausea and vomiting and analgesics for myalgia can also be administered (Nguyen 2018).

Contact isolation is required for hospitalized patients with rotavirus. Patients should be in a single room with a dedicated toilet and equipment. Healthcare professionals should use PPE for contact isolation. Contact precautions should be continued throughout the duration of the illness (CDC 2019; Nguyen 2018).

Parvovirus B19

Parvovirus B19, also known as erythema infectiosum or Fifth disease, is a virus of the Parvoviridae family which only affects humans. Many other parvovirus strains have an effect on animals. Although some individuals for parvovirus B19 may be asymptomatic, oftentimes symptoms are vague. Fever, headache, myalgia, malaise, nausea, and rhinorrhea are common symptoms, seen within the first 7 days after infection. A bright red macular exanthem of the cheeks, circumoral pallor, and atypical or maculopapular rash can occur. Parvovirus 19 is also associated with aplastic crisis. Hydrops fetalis may result in pregnant women who contract parvovirus 19 (Cennimo 2019).

Management of parvovirus 19 is mainly supportive, focusing on the symptoms. Antipyretics may be given for fever, and intravenous immunoglobulin (IVIG) may be used in patients with red-cell aplasia. Patients in aplastic crisis will need red blood cell transfusions (Cennimo 2019).

Precautions for patients with parvovirus 19 include droplet plus standard. When chronic disease occurs in a patient who is immunocompromised, precautions are maintained for the duration of the hospitalization. A patient with transient aplastic crisis or red-cell crisis should have these precautions maintained for 7 days (CDC 2019).

Rubeola (Measles)

Rubeola, or measles, is caused by the measles virus which is an RNA virus of the Morbillivirus. Although not as common as it was previously due to vaccinations, measles is still seen in patients who are not yet vaccinated, are immunocompromised, or have lost passive immunity. It is a highly contagious virus, spread through droplet or contact with secretions (Chen 2019).

Measles is generally managed with supportive care and infrequently leads to hospitalization. Hydration, fluid management, and vitamin supplementation are strategies. Antiviral therapy may also be considered. Hospitalization may occur with secondary complications, such as pneumonia, dehydration, superinfections, or croup. Secondary infections will need treatment with antibiotics (Chen 2019).

Patients hospitalized with measles require airborne isolation and precautions in a single, negative-pressure room when communicable. Measles is considered communicable around 3–5 days before a rash appears to approximately 4 days after rash appearance. Patients who are immunocompromised should be isolated throughout the course of the illness (CDC 2019; Chen 2019). It is recommended that healthcare professionals who have had vaccinations or are previously immune to measles be assigned to care for these patients (CDC 2019).

Rubella

Rubella, also known as the German measles or 3-day measles, is actually a completely different disease than measles. The rubivirus which causes the disease is highly contagious. Although not as common as it was previously due to vaccinations, rubella is still seen in patients who are not yet vaccinated, are immunocompromised, or have lost passive immunity. It is spread through droplet or contact with secretions (The College of Physicians of Philadelphia 2019).

Children with rubella tend to have mild symptoms, with generally a low-grade fever, sore throat, myalgia, eye pain, and respiratory symptoms. A pink or light red rash appears, usually within 2–3 weeks of exposure. Rubella is contagious for 5–21 days, including prior to the onset of rash. Adults are more susceptible to complications, such as neuritis, encephalitis, and arthritis (Ezike 2017; The College of Physicians of Philadelphia 2019). If rubella is contracted during pregnancy then the fetus or neonate can be affected (see congenital rubella).

Management of rubella is generally supportive, including fluids and medications to reduce fever. Patients in hospital with rubella require isolation with droplet and standard precautions. Isolation should continue until 7 days after the onset of rash. Healthcare professionals who are susceptible to rubella should not enter the room if immune team members are available. If a healthcare worker is exposed and is susceptible, rubella vaccination should be given within 3 days of exposure (for individuals who are not pregnant). This personnel should also be quarantined from days 5–21, regardless of if vaccination was given. Nonimmune pregnant women should not care for rubella patients (CDC 2019).

Congenital Rubella

Fetal exposure to the rubivirus, especially during the first trimester, can lead to congenital rubella, also known as congenital rubella syndrome (CRS). Maternal rubella infection can affect the fetus, and the effects are at their greatest during the first 12–14 weeks of pregnancy. Miscarriages and stillbirths may occur. If exposure occurs after 20 weeks, the likelihood of neonatal complications is much lower (Ezike 2017; Lanzieri et al. 2020).

For infants born with congenital rubella syndrome, there are multiple complications that may occur. Congenital cataracts or glaucoma, hearing impairment, and congenital heart disease (such as patent ductus arteriosus or pulmonary stenosis) are most commonly seen with congenital rubella syndrome. Other symptoms may include purpura, pigmentary retinopathy, hepatosplenomegaly, hyperbilirubinemia, microcephaly, meningoencephalitis, bone disease, or developmental delays (Ezike 2017; Lanzieri et al. 2020).

Management of congenital rubella syndrome is supportive and focused on the complications. Neonates require hearing and vision screening. An ophthalmologist should evaluate the eyes. Interventions for hyperbilirubinemia, such as phototherapy and exchange transfusions, may be needed. An echocardiogram should be performed to assess for heart defects. If present, monitoring for congestive heart failure is necessary (Ezike 2017; Lanzieri et al. 2020).

Infants with congenital rubella syndrome may remain contagious for up to 1 year. When in hospital, contact isolation plus standard precautions are required. It is recommended to keep this isolation in place up until 1 year of age unless nasopharyngeal and urine cultures are negative after 3 months of age. At that time, only standard precautions in hospital are needed (CDC 2019; Lanzieri et al. 2020).

Infectious Parotitis (Mumps)

Infectious parotitis, also known as mumps, is caused by an RNA virus known as rubulavirus. The viral infection affects the salivary glands, particularly the parotid gland. Transmission is through droplets, saliva, and contact, with an incubation period of 12–25 days following exposure. Incidence of mumps has decreased with the use of vaccinations. Symptoms include enlargement of the salivary and parotid glands, fever, headache, earache, and malaise. Thyroiditis may occur, and pancreatitis is a rare effect (Defendi 2019).

Management of mumps is supportive, with antipyretics for fever, analgesics for pain, hydration, and warm or cold packs for comfort (Defendi 2019). In hospital, patients with mumps require droplet plus standard precautions. Isolation should continue until 5 days after the onset of swelling. Healthcare professionals who are susceptible should not care for these patients if immune staff are available (CDC 2019).

Varicella (Chickenpox)

Varicella, also known as chickenpox, is caused by the varicella zoster virus, a double-stranded deoxyribonucleic acid virus. It is spread through airborne droplets and contact with the vesicles that appear during the course of illness. Like measles, incidence of chickenpox has decreased with the increased use of vaccinations (Papadopoulos 2020).

Management of chickenpox is mainly supportive, focusing on the treatment of pruritis with oral or topical agents. In patients who are immunocompromised, acyclovir therapy is recommended. Secondary infections may occur with cutaneous lesions, including the development of pneumonia or meningitis. Antibiotics are required to treat bacterial infections (Papadopoulos 2020).

If a patient is hospitalized with varicella, they require airborne isolation and precautions in a single, negative-pressure room when communicable. Chickenpox is considered communicable about 1–3 days before lesions appear until all lesions have crusted, or no new lesions develop. Patients who are immunocompromised should be isolated throughout the course of the illness (CDC 2021b; Papadopoulos 2020). It is recommended that healthcare professionals who have had vaccinations or are previously immune to varicella be assigned to care for these patients (CDC 2019).

Herpes Zoster (Varicella Zoster, or Shingles)

Herpes zoster is also known as varicella zoster or shingles. This viral infection is a result of a reactivation of the varicella zoster virus, often decades after an individual has been exposed to varicella. It is estimated that over 95% of adults over 40 have antibodies to varicella zoster virus, and are at risk for reactivation of the virus. The incidence is beginning to decrease since introduction of the vaccination for varicella and now for varicella zoster (Janniger 2021).

Symptoms of herpes zoster may start with general unwellness, including fever and anorexia. Shingles causes a self-limiting rash along one or more dermatomes, which lasts from 1 to 10 days. Pain is the most common symptom of the rash, but pruritis and numbness may also be present. Erythema, lymphadenopathy, and vesicle formation also occur. Postherpetic neuralgia (PHN) is pain in the dermatome(s) that lasts for months to years, even after the resolution of the rash and vesicles (Janniger 2021).

Management of herpes zoster depends on the severity of the illness as well as the immune state of the individual affected. Non-steroidal anti-inflammatory medication, wet dressings, and calamine lotion may be used. Patients with severe infections, those who are elderly, or who are immunocompromised may be treated with steroids, analgesics, anticonvulsants, and antiviral agents. Hospitalization may be concerned in cases of disseminated herpes zoster, severe symptoms or involvement of more than two dermatomes, immunosuppression, atypical presentations (such as myelitis), facial bacterial superinfection, or involvement of an ophthalmic or meningoencephalopathic nature (Janniger 2021). Patients who are admitted with disseminated disease, require airborne isolation plus contact precautions for the duration of the illness. Immunocompromised patients admitted with localized disease require airborne isolation and contact precautions until they are ruled out for disseminated disease. If the herpes zoster infection is localized in a patient with an intact immune system, and has lesions that can be contained and covered, then standard precautions are used until the lesions are dry and crusted. Healthcare professionals who are susceptible to varicella should not enter the room or provide direct patient care if immune caregivers are available (CDC 2019).

Influenza

Influenza, known commonly as the flu, is a highly contagious viral disease that is transmitted via aerosol from one person to another. The incubation period for influenza ranges from 1 to 4 days and may be contagious prior to the onset of symptoms. There are different forms of influenza, including influenza A and B, and avian influenza. It is estimated that up to 62,000 deaths occurred from influenza during the 2019–2020 season. With the emergence of COVID 19, it is difficult for accurate statistics. Signs and symptoms may include fever, myalgia, sore throat, headache, weakness and fatigue, nasal discharge, cough or other respiratory symptoms, tachycardia, and reddened eyes. Diagnosis is based on clinical presentation and can be confirmed through rapid influenza testing (Nguyen 2021).

Prevention of influenza is vital, due to its high risk for spread. Mortality is greatest in vulnerable populations, such as the elderly and infants. Vaccinations against influenza A and B should be administered each year before flu season. The CDC makes changes to the seasonal vaccination subtypes every year, based on international trends (Nguyen 2021).

Management of patients with influenza depends on the severity of the infection, including signs and symptoms. Generally, supportive care is given, such as oral fluids, rest, and antipyretics if needed. Some patients may need oxygen, intravenous fluids, or even ventilatory support if there is respiratory failure. The use of antiviral medication may also be indicated, such as baloxavir marboxil, oseltamivir, peramivir, and zanamivir (Nguyen 2021). For hospitalized patients with seasonal or avian influenza, standard precautions are all that is needed. If there is a novel influenza A strain associated with severe illness, or pandemic influenza, then droplet plus standard precautions should be utilized (CDC 2019).

Respiratory Syncytial Virus (RSV)

Respiratory syncytial virus, or RSV, is the main cause of bronchiolitis in pediatric patients, which many times require acute inpatient hospital stays. RSV infections can also cause hospitalizations in elderly patients. It is estimated that up to five million children under the age of 4 in the United States acquire an RSV infection each year, with more than 125,000 of these cases requiring hospitalization. And in elderly patients over the age of 65 in the United States, over 175,000 are hospitalized with RSV and approximately 14,000 die from the infection (Krilov 2019). Signs and symptoms of RSV include upper respiratory tract infection, including cough, retractions, wheezing, rales, tachypnea, apnea (with infants), and cyanosis, as well as fever (Krilov 2019).

Prevention of RSV transmission is critical, particularly with high-risk neonates and infants, such as those born premature. The

American Academy of Pediatrics (AAP) has provided guidelines for the administration of RSV prophylaxis with the medication palivizumab. The recommendations include infants younger than 24 months who have hemodynamically significant congenital heart disease or chronic lung disease and are off oxygen or pulmonary medications for less than 6 months at the start of the RSV season; premature infants born at 28 weeks' gestational age or less who are younger than 1 year chronologically at the start of the RSV season; premature infants born at 29–32 weeks' gestational age who are younger than 6 months old chronologically at the start of the RSV season; and infants born at 32–35 weeks' gestational age who are younger than 3 months old chronologically age at the start of or during the RSV season have high exposure risk (Krilov 2019).

Management of RSV is mainly supportive, including hydration and oxygen as needed. Many pediatric patients may need intravenous therapy for hydration, due to vomiting of milk or feedings. The use of bronchodilators, epinephrine, and corticosteroids may occur, although there is limited evidence to demonstrate the effectiveness of these medications. The antiviral agent ribavirin may be given aerosolized in severe cases (Krilov 2019). For hospitalized patients with RSV, contact plus standard precautions should be used, including a mask if there is a potential to come in contact with splash (CDC 2019).

Acute Viral Conjunctivitis

Acute viral conjunctivitis, also known as pink eye, is the result of a condition usually caused by adenovirus. Herpes simplex, varicella zoster, picornavirus, poxvirus, and human immunodeficiency virus may also cause acute viral conjunctivitis. Viral conjunctivitis is highly contagious as long as the eyes are red, which can be from 10 to 14 days. Transmission occurs through viral particles from patient contact, infected respiratory droplets, fomites, or contaminated water sources (such as swimming pools). Patients with pink eye should avoid touching their eyes, shaking hands, or sharing towels, napkins, pillowcases, etc., among other activities. The conjunctivitis infection is self-limiting, generally resolving within 2–4 weeks. Signs and symptoms of acute viral conjunctivitis are itchy, watery eyes, redness, discharge, and sensitivity to light (Scott 2020).

Management of acute viral conjunctivitis is supportive. Cold compresses and lubricants may be used to decrease discomfort. For patients who are susceptible to superinfection, a topical antibacterial may be used in the eyes. Topical antiviral medication may also be given if the causative virus is known (Scott 2020). Patients with acute viral conjunctivitis who are hospitalized required contact and standard precautions for the duration of the illness. With the highly contagious nature of this infection, outbreaks may occur in communities, clinics, and in neonatal and pediatric settings. Diligence is needed to prevent the spread (CDC 2019).

Diphtheria

Corynebacterium diphtheria is an aerobic gram-positive bacterium which can cause an upper respiratory or cutaneous infection. Onset of symptoms usually appear within 2–5 days of exposure, but diphtheria can be contagious for 2–6 weeks if antibiotic treatment is not started. Individuals can be susceptible to the infection if they have not been vaccinated or have impaired immunity. Respiratory symptoms generally include sore throat, pharyngeal inflammation, cervical adenopathy, and development of pseudomembrane in the respiratory tract, with mucosa that is bleeding and edematous. Cutaneous diphtheria symptoms include nonhealing ulcers that are covered with a gray membrane, which often have a coinfection, such as staphylococcus aureus and group A streptococci. Other symptoms of diphtheria include fever, malaise, weakness, headache, dysphagia, nasal discharge, dyspnea, wheezing, stridor, and cough (Lo 2019).

Diphtheria is associated with high mortality due to respiratory compromise. Airways must be maintained, and intubation may be necessary. Antibiotic therapy should be immediately established, and diphtheria antitoxin may be administered in severe cases.

Fluid maintenance and monitoring for cardiac arrhythmias are also important. Management of pharyngeal diphtheria includes use of droplet plus standard precautions, while the use of contact plus standard precautions is recommended for cutaneous diphtheria. If patients have a combination, then droplet, contact, and standard precautions should all be used. Precautions should continue until the patient is finished with antimicrobial treatment, and two cultures taken 24 h apart are negative (CDC 2019; Lo 2019).

Pertussis (Whooping Cough)

Pertussis, also known as whooping cough, is an infection of the respiratory tract, usually caused by Bordetella pertussis (occasionally Bordetella parapertussis). Although there has been a significant decrease in cases with effective immunizations, there are still outbreaks that occur. Pertussis is associated with high morbidity and mortality in pediatric patients under the age of two. Pertussis is highly contagious, with an incubation period of approximately 3–12 days. The disease itself typically lasts for 6 weeks, consisting of three stages that last 1–2 weeks. The first phase is known as the catarrhal phase, in which symptoms appear similar to a cold or flu, such as rhinorrhea, nasal congestion, sneezing, low-grade fever, and eye tearing. The second phase is the paroxysmal phase, where paroxysms of coughing, often over several minutes, occur. After this intense coughing, often a loud whoop can be heard related to air attempting to be inhaled through obstructed airways. Incidences of apnea and exhaustion are seen after paroxysms of coughing, particularly in infants. Reddened face and vomiting may also occur. The last stage of pertussis is the convalescent phase, which is a chronic cough (Bocka 2019).

Infants, immunocompromised, or patients with moderate to severe pertussis are often hospitalized for respiratory support and monitoring, at times required intensive care. Management includes oxygen, bronchodilators, antibiotics, fluids, and nutrition. Intubation and ventilation may be needed in severe cases. Patients are placed in droplet plus standard precautions until

5 days after initiating effective antibiotic therapy (Bocka 2019; CDC 2019).

Viral Hepatitis

Hepatitis is a general term that describes inflammation of the liver, which may be a result of infection or noninfectious causes. Viral hepatitis is responsible for over half of the hepatitis cases that occur in the United States (Samji 2017). Viral hepatitis is caused by a number of viruses, but most commonly are hepatitis A virus (HAV), hepatitis B virus (HBV), and hepatitis C virus (HCV). Hepatitis D and E are not as common. Viral hepatitis can either be acute or chronic. Patients may be asymptomatic or mildly symptomatic, or may quickly progress to liver failure. Signs and symptoms can include anorexia, nausea, vomiting, alterations in taste, arthralgias, malaise, fatigue, urticaria, pruritus, dark urine, pale stools, upper abdominal pain, icterus, abnormal liver enzymes, encephalopathy, and hepatomegaly (Samji 2017).

Management of viral hepatitis includes supportive care, such as fluid and electrolyte management, antiemetics, and monitoring. If admitted to hospital, patients with viral hepatitis generally require standard precautions only. With patients who have type A or type E hepatitis and use diapers or are incontinent, contact plus standard precautions are recommended (CDC 2019; Samji 2017).

Herpes Simplex

Herpes simplex, also known as herpesvirus hominis, has two types: herpes simplex virus type 1 (HSV-1) is generally associated with orofacial disease; type 2 herpes simplex virus (HSV-2) is connected with genital disease. The locations of the lesions do not necessarily indicate the viral type of herpes simplex. The virus is transmitted through bodily fluids, such as saliva, with an incubation period of less than 1 week. Many times, herpes simplex is asymptomatic and can be a primary or recurrent infection. Symptoms, including systemic signs, can be prolonged and cause complications, particularly in immunocompromised patients. The manifestation of herpes simplex virus can also cause different signs and symptoms, many times lasting a few weeks. Symptoms of acute herpetic gingivostomatitis include fever, anorexia, fatigue, gingivitis, oral vesicular lesions, lymphadenopathy, and perioral skin involvement. Symptoms of acute herpetic pharyngo-tonsillitis include tonsillitis, pharyngitis, fever, malaise, headache, sore throat, and lesions on tonsil and pharynx. Herpes labialis, also known as cold sores, has symptoms including pain, burning, and tingling at the affected site (usually around the lips), and pustular vesicles that ulcerate. Genital herpes is mainly transmitted via oral to genital contact, with symptoms of fever, headache, malaise, myalgia, pain and itching at the affected site, dysuria, vaginal and urethral discharge, lymphadenopathy, and herpetic vesicles on the external genitalia. Complications of herpes simplex consist of disseminated infection, pneumonitis, hepatitis, or meningoencephalitis (Ayoade 2021).

Management of herpes simplex includes the use of antiviral medications, specified for the site and manifestation of the virus. Use of standard precautions are recommended for most patients who have herpes simplex while hospitalized. Contact plus standard precautions are recommended if a patient has severe disseminated or primary mucocutaneous herpes simplex until lesions are dry and crusted over. Neonatal patients with lesions or exposure to herpes simplex during delivery should also be placed in contact plus standard precautions until lesions are dry and crusted, or surface cultures are obtained (CDC 2019; Ayoade 2021).

Lice

Lice are parasites that live in the body, by feeding on human blood. Lice pierce the skin and inject saliva to obtain the blood, which oftentimes cause pruritis. A mature female louse lays about three to six white eggs a day, known as nits. After approximately 9 days, the eggs hatch and the louse can live for 30–45 days. There

are different species of lice which prefer to feed on various locations on the host's body. Pediculus capitis is also known as head
lice. Pediculus corporis is also referred to as body lice. Pthirus
pubis is also known as pubic lice or often called "crabs." Symptoms
of lice include pruritis (often intense), evidence of bites (such as
wheals or papules), excoriations (from scratching), and lymphadenopathy. The examination of a patient shows visible lice and
nits in the hair of the affected area (Guenther 2019).

Management of lice depends on the type and location of the
infestation. Pediculicides are medications to treat and get rid of
lice, which can be ovicidal or non-ovicidal to kill the nits. Manual
removal of nits may be done in combination with a pediculicide.
Material that may be potentially contaminated, including clothing, bedding, hats, scarves, towels, and stuffed animals should be
washed in hot water and dried in a hot setting in the dryer. If items
cannot be machine washed, then dry-cleaning, or sealing and stor-
ing in a plastic bag for 2 weeks is recommended. Hair items such
as brushes, combs, and hair accessories should be disposed of and
replaced, or sealed and stored in a plastic bag for 2 weeks. If a
patient who is hospitalized has a body or pubic lice, then standard
precautions are recommended. For those patients with head lice,
contact and standard precautions are recommended until 24 h of
initiation of effective therapy. Staff who remove patient's clothing
should wear gown and gloves, and immediately bag the garments
for machine washing (CDC 2019; Guenther 2019).

Meningitis

Meningitis is when there is an inflammation of the meninges, usually caused by bacterial or viral infections. An infectious agent
from local infection or colonization can spread to the central nervous system and affect the meninges. Most common is invasion of
the bloodstream, which is seen in meningococcal, cryptococcal,
syphilitic, and pneumococcal meningitis. Common signs and
symptoms of meningitis are known as the triad, which include
fever, headache, and neck stiffness. Altered mental status, nausea,
vomiting, sleepiness, fatigue, myalgia, and photophobia are other

symptoms. Infants with meningitis may have a bulging fontanelle, paradoxic irritability, hypotonia, and a high-pitched cry (Vasudeva 2021).

Management of meningitis depends on the cause, type of organism involved, and severity of symptoms. Stabilization may be required in acute cases, including fluid management, crystalloids, oxygen, and treatment of seizures. Monitoring, seizure precautions, correction of electrolyte imbalances, and treatment of comorbidity exacerbations may also be required. Antibiotics are required for bacterial meningitis, beginning with empirical antibiotics and then targeted antibiotics once the organism is identified. Antiviral medications may be needed to treat viral meningitis. Other types of meningitis may need treatment based on the identified pathogen, such as antifungals, for example. Precautions and isolation for patients hospitalized with meningitis are based on the cause of the infection. Standard precautions are recommended for meningitis caused by fungi, gram-negative bacteria, listeria monocytogenes, and streptococcus pneumoniae. If an enterovirus infection is present, then contact plus standard precautions are endorsed for diapered or incontinent patients. Droplet plus standard precautions are recommended until 24 h after effective therapy is initiated for meningitis caused by known or suspected type B haemophilus influenzae, neisseria meningitidis, and meningococcal disease with sepsis or pneumonia. For meningitis caused by M. tuberculosis contact and/or airborne precautions may be necessary if there is active pulmonary disease, draining cutaneous lesions, or pediatric patients (until family members are ruled out) (CDC 2019; Vasudeva 2021).

Tuberculosis (TB)

Tuberculosis (TB) is caused by the organism M tuberculosis, which is an aerobe and intracellular parasite. Although TB is generally associated with the lungs, the M tuberculosis organism can spread to the lymph system, organs (including spleen, liver, kidneys, and brain), bones, and bone marrow. The organism is primarily spread through airborne methods by patients infected with TB (Herchline 2020).

Management of TB includes the use of a medication regimen of four drugs. These include isoniazid, rifampin, pyrazinamide, and the addition of either ethambutol or streptomycin. Medications are reevaluated after 2 months, and course of treatment is typically 6 months in duration. Patients should have sputum analyzed during treatment to assess for conversion of M tuberculosis. Toxicity monitoring for medications is also necessary including complete blood count, liver enzymes, and serum creatinine levels (Herchline 2020).

Infectious patients with TB require airborne isolation in a single, negative-pressure room. In addition to contact precautions, healthcare professionals require the use of either N95 masks or PAPRs when working with TB patients. Isolation should be continued for approximately 2–4 weeks, until sputum samples are negative for three consecutive results (CDC 2019; Herchline 2020).

Rhinoviruses

There are over 200 different antigenically distinct forms of rhinoviruses, also known as the common cold. These viruses are from the Picornaviridae family, and it is estimated that each person has three to six cases of the common cold every year in the United States. Rhinoviruses cause upper respiratory tract infections and may exacerbate chronic respiratory conditions, such as asthma, chronic obstructive pulmonary disease (COPD), and cystic fibrosis. The incubation period for rhinoviruses ranges from 12 to 72 h, with symptoms lasting from 7–14 days. Symptoms include rhinorrhea, nasal congestion, sneezing, sore throat, coughing, and headache. Low-grade fever may be seen in children less than 5 years of age (Buensalido 2019).

Management of rhinovirus is mainly symptom control, as the infection is usually mild and self-limiting. Support is rest, hydration, antihistamines, and nasal decongestants. If a patient who is hospitalized develops a rhinovirus then droplet plus standard precautions are recommended for the duration of the illness. If a patient has copious secretions, then the addition of contact precautions is suggested. Outbreaks of rhinoviruses have occurred in neonatal intensive care units and long-term care facilities. These vulnerable patients are at higher risk for complications (Buensalido 2019; CDC 2019).

References

Ayoade, F. (2021). Herpes simplex. https://emedicine.medscape.com/article/218580-overview

Bocka, J. (2019). Pertussis. https://emedicine.medscape.com/article/967268-overview

Buensalido, J. (2019). Rhinovirus (RV) infection (common cold). https://emedicine.medscape.com/article/227820-overview

Bush, M., & Vazquez-Pertejo, M. (2021). Staphylococcal infections. Merck Manual. https://www.merckmanuals.com/professional/infectious-diseases/gram-positive-cocci/staphylococcal-infections

Centers for Disease Control & Prevention. (2017). Management of multidrug-resistant organisms in healthcare settings, 2006 (updated 2017). https://www.cdc.gov/infectioncontrol/pdf/guidelines/mdro-guidelines.pdf

Centers for Disease Control & Prevention. (2019). 2007 guideline for isolation precautions: Preventing transmission of infectious agents in healthcare settings (updated 2019). https://www.cdc.gov/infectioncontrol/pdf/guidelines/isolation-guidelines-H.pdf

Centers for Disease Control & Prevention. (2021a). About COVID 19. https://www.cdc.gov/coronavirus/2019-ncov/your-health/about-covid-19.html

Centers for Disease Control & Prevention. (2021b). Chickenpox (varicella) for healthcare professionals. https://www.cdc.gov/chickenpox/hcp/index.html

Chen, S. (2019). Measles. https://emedicine.medscape.com/article/966220-overview#a5

Cennimo, D. (2019). Parvovirus B19 infection. https://emedicine.medscape.com/article/961063-overview

Defendi, G. (2019). Mumps. https://reference.medscape.com/article/966678-overview

Ezike, E. (2017). Pediatric rubella clinical presentation. https://emedicine.medscape.com/article/968523-clinical

Grinspan, A. (2021). C. difficile infection. American College of Gastroenterology. https://gi.org/topics/c-difficile-infection/

Guenther, L. (2019). Pediculosis and pthiriasis (lice infestation). https://emedicine.medscape.com/article/225013-overview

Herchline, T. (2020). Tuberculosis (TB). https://emedicine.medscape.com/article/230802-overview

Janniger, C. (2021). Herpes zoster. https://emedicine.medscape.com/article/1132465-overview

Khan, Z. (2018). Norovirus. https://emedicine.medscape.com/article/224225-overview

Khan, Z. (2021). Group A streptococcus (GAS) infections. https://emedicine.medscape.com/article/228936-overview

Krilov, L. (2019). Respiratory syncytial virus infection. https://emedicine.medscape.com/article/971488-overview

Lanzieri, T., Redd, S., Abernathy, E., & Icenogle, J. (2020). *Manual for the surveillance of vaccine-preventable diseases: Chapter 15: Congenital rubella syndrome*. https://www.cdc.gov/vaccines/pubs/surv-manual/chpt15-crs.html

Lo, B. (2019). Diphtheria. https://emedicine.medscape.com/article/782051-overview

National Institutes of Health. (2021). COVID-19 treatment guidelines. https://www.covid19treatmentguidelines.nih.gov

Nguyen, D. (2018). Rotavirus. https://emedicine.medscape.com/article/803885-overview#a4

Nguyen, H. (2021). Influenza. https://emedicine.medscape.com/article/219557-overview

Papadakis, M.A., McPhee, S.J., & Bernstein, J. (Eds.), (2020). *Quick medical diagnosis & treatment 2020*. McGraw Hill.

Papadopoulos, A. (2020). Chickenpox. https://emedicine.medscape.com/article/1131785-overview

Samji, N. (2017). Viral hepatitis. https://emedicine.medscape.com/article/775507-overview

Scott, I. (2020). Viral conjunctivitis (pink eye). https://emedicine.medscape.com/article/1191370-overview

Taylor, T.A., & Unakal, C.G. (2021). Staphylococcus aureus. In: StatPearls https://www.ncbi.nlm.nih.gov/books/NBK441868/

The College of Physicians of Philadelphia. (2019). Rubella. https://www.historyofvaccines.org/content/articles/rubella

Vasudeva, S. (2021). Meningitis. https://emedicine.medscape.com/article/232915-overview

Types of Errors

3

Medical errors are the cause of almost 9.5% of all deaths annually in the United States (Institute of Medicine 2000; Johns Hopkins Medicine 2016). These include medication errors, hospital-acquired infections, and accidents, such as falls, to name a few. Nurses play a key role in the prevention of errors, and unfortunately, they also play a key role in making errors. Many errors are due to poor processes or failure to follow policies and procedures. You get what you plan for; therefore, if you have poor outcomes, you should probably start looking at the processes that contribute to the poor outcomes.: If you have weak processes and then throw inpatient complications, such as COVID 19, you will most likely increase your risk of errors and poor outcomes.

Errors Associated with Isolation and Precautions

When working with infectious patients, most errors occur with precautions compliance. Hand hygiene compliance has been noted in studies to be as low as 50% in acute care settings. During the COVID 19 pandemic, some hand hygiene compliance rates were seen as high as 88–98% in 2020 and then declined once again. The number of hand hygiene opportunities was negatively

© The Author(s), under exclusive license to Springer Nature Switzerland AG 2022
K. Maryniak, R. Garrett, *Preventing Errors and Pitfalls in Nursing with Infectious Patients*, https://doi.org/10.1007/978-3-030-86728-7_3

correlated with hand hygiene compliance; meaning that the more opportunities there were, the less observed hand hygiene performance was noted (Makini et al. 2021).

Compliance with appropriate use of PPE, including donning and doffing, was also noted to be low in studies. Studies have discussed 52–70% full compliance with contact precautions in hospitals, including only 7–22% with C. diff patients. There were descriptions of only 34% compliance of healthcare professionals with required PPE for droplet precautions. Only 17–50% of professionals removed PPE in the correct sequence and properly disposed of it prior to leaving the isolation room (Krein et al. 2018).

Observational studies describe PPE noncompliance. One type of noncompliance with the use of PPE is known as a violation, in which standard practices or policies are not followed. Observations of violation include not donning appropriate PPE, improper or incomplete use of PPE, and doffing or disposal of used PPE outside of the patient room. Some violations were noted where the healthcare professional did not intend to have contact with the patient or environment but unknowingly did expose themselves. Violations were also noted with urgent or emergent care, in which the precautions were not followed due to the need to provide immediate care. Other violations were demonstrations of reckless behavior in which the healthcare professional knowingly violated precautions even with direct contact with the patient or environment (Krein et al. 2018).

Mistakes are other errors observed with PPE, particularly with doffing. These failures expose healthcare professionals to contamination. This includes improper techniques for doffing or failure to follow the appropriate sequence for taking off PPE. Other mistakes have been observed based on situations which can increase risk for self-contamination. Examples include using contaminated gloves to touch items such as pens, badges, or stethoscopes without cleaning afterward (Krein et al. 2018).

Slips occurred as well with the use of PPE, which are based on automatic behaviors. Examples include touching hair, face, or phone with contaminated gloves. These slips are unconscious and the person is not even aware of the action (Krein et al. 2018).

Errors Related to Hospital-Acquired Conditions and Falls

Although not all patient harm is associated with errors, some errors can result in hospital-acquired conditions or falls. Nurses commonly perform what is referred to as "stacking." Stacking is when there are multiple cognitive processes and competing priorities in the mind. The ability to manage many plans and thoughts for carrying outpatient care through stacking can be impeded by the environment, changing situations, interruptions, delays, or time constraints. The practice environment consists of work design, supportive staffing (which includes skill mix as well as the number of staff), organizational management (which can impact policies, assignments, and resources), and the culture of the work environment (Al-ghraiybah et al. 2021; Thomas et al. 2017).

Hospital-acquired conditions (HACs) include central line-associated bloodstream infections (CLABSIs), catheter-associated urinary tract infections (CAUTIs), venous thromboembolism (VTE), ventilator-associated events (VAEs) pressure injuries, and hospital-acquired infections (also referred to as nosocomial infections). Preventable falls in hospitals can also occur.

Errors that can contribute to hospital-acquired conditions or falls include lack of timely or appropriate assessment. Assessment can be interrupted, delayed, or missed, due to the practice environment or issues affecting cognitive stacking (Al-ghraiybah et al. 2021; Roth et al. 2017; Thomas et al. 2017). Fall risk, VTE risk, and skin assessments are required frequently. Patients on ventilators should be assessed at least daily for continuation. Assessment of lines and drains are also necessary on a consistent basis. Missed assessments can lead to increased risk for falls, pressure injuries, CLABSIs, and CAUTIs. Delayed or missing assessments of peripheral intravenous (IV) sites may also lead to infiltration or extravasation from medication administration.

Delays, missed care opportunities, or not performing interventions can also occur, which are errors that can predispose patients to hospital-acquired conditions or falls (Al-ghraiybah et al. 2021; Roth et al. 2017; Thomas et al. 2017). Examples can be lack of catheter care or perineal care for patients with indwelling urinary catheters, which can lead to CAUTIs. Inappropriate cleaning or central line access can create chance of CLABSIs. Failure to provide appropriate oral care can contribute to the development of ventilator-associated pneumonia (VAP). Lack of turning patients or using appropriate mattresses can increase risk of pressure injuries. Missing strategies for fall prevention, particularly for patients at high risk, can lead to avoidable falls. Inadequate or missing interventions for VTE prophylaxis can create risk for VTE development.

Failures in communication, both written and verbal, can also create errors (Roth et al. 2017; Thomas et al. 2017). Verbal communication mainly occurs with reports and handoffs. Using checklists and standardized tools to provide verbal communication can create more complete reports and ensure that vital patient information is passed along. Examples of communication tools may be SBAR or I-PASS (Miller 2021; Roth et al. 2017). See also Chap. 6. Additionally, providing a bedside report with the off-going nurse, the oncoming nurse, and the patient (and family, if able). Effective bedside report can ensure that there is a verbal and visual handoff, which can increase patient safety (Bigani and Correia 2018).

Complete documentation of assessment, interventions, and nursing care planning is essential. Fall risk assessments should be done real time, and risk assessment scores will vary with changes in patient condition. The same is true of skin assessments and risks for pressure injury, as well as VTE risk assessments. Documentation of lines and drains must be clear as well (Maryniak 2021). Even with complete documentation, nurses caring for patients must read what is charted and apply it. An important consideration to assist with critical thinking is looking for trends in patient care status. Identifying and applying trends is helpful in proactively planning and intervening on behalf of the patient (Maryniak 2021).

Errors Associated with Restraints

In the United States, the use of restraints must follow Centers for Medicaid & Medicare Services (CMS) rules (2020). Restraints can include physical restraints or chemical restraints for violent or nonviolent behavior. Common errors include lack of provider order for initiating or continuing restraints or specific provider orders for restraints. Lack of understanding of restraint requirements is frequently seen, such as indications, alternatives, and types of restraints. Missed assessments and observation requirements are also sources of errors. Additionally, knowledge gaps surrounding patient rights and restraints have been seen as lacking (Lee et al. 2021).

Medication Errors

It is difficult to quantify how many medication errors occur as there is no centralized reporting system for all errors. Some studies show that medication errors can occur between 32 and 94% of the time, with 38% of those errors attributed to nursing (Salar et al. 2020). The most common medication errors by nursing are wrong dose, wrong time, omissions, and wrong medication (MacDowell et al. 2021).

Just as previously discussed, there are multiple contributing factors, which can lead to medication errors. Slips and lapses were identified in studies as a common cause of medication errors. Communications, supplies, and inadequate processes also contributed. Personal factors, as well as system features, can create high risk for medication errors (Maryniak 2016, 2018).

References

Al-ghraiybah, T., Sim, J., & Lago, L. (2021). The relationship between the nursing practice environment and five nursing-sensitive patient outcomes in acute care hospitals: A systematic review. *Nursing Open, 8*(5), 2262-2271.

Bigani, D. K., & Correia, A. M. (2018). On the same page: Nurse, patient, and family perceptions of change-of-shift bedside report. *Journal of Pediatric Nursing, 41*, 84–89.

Centers for Medicare & Medicaid Services (CMS). (2020). *State operations manual: Appendix A: Survey protocol, regulations and interpretive guidelines for hospitals.* https://www.cms.gov/Regulations-and-Guidance/Guidance/Manuals/Downloads/som107ap_a_hospitals.pdf

Institute of Medicine. (2000). *To err is human: Building a safer health system*. National Academies Press.

Johns Hopkins Medicine. (2016). Study suggests medical errors now third leading cause of death in the U.S. https://www.hopkinsmedicine.org/news/media/releases

Krein, S. L., Mayer, J., Harrod, M., Weston, L. E., Gregory, L., Petersen, L., Samore, M. H., & Drews, F. A. (2018). Identification and characterization of failures in infectious agent transmission precaution practices in hospitals: A qualitative study. *JAMA Internal Medicine, 178*(8), 1016–1057.

Lee, T.-K., Välimäki, M., & Lantta, T. (2021). The knowledge, practice and attitudes of nurses regarding physical restraint: Survey results from psychiatric inpatient settings. *International Journal of Environmental Research and Public Health, 18*(13).

MacDowell, P., Cabri, A., & Davis, M. (2021). Medication administration errors. Patient Safety Network. https://psnet.ahrq.gov/primer/medication-administration-errors

Makini, S., Umschied, C., Soo, J., Chu, V., Barlett, A., Landon, E., & Marrs, R. (2021). Hand hygiene compliance rate during the COVID-19 pandemic. *JAMA Internal Medicine, 181*(7), 1006-1008.

Maryniak, K. (2016). How to avoid medication errors in nursing. https://www.rn.com/nursing-news/nurses-role-in-medication-error-prevention/

Maryniak, K. (2018). *Medication errors: Best practices for prevention* (webinar). Lorman.

Maryniak, K. (2021). *Documentation for nurses* (4th ed.) (ebook). Elite Healthcare.

Miller, D. (2021). I-PASS as a nursing communication tool. *Pediatric Nursing, 47*(1), 30–37.

Roth, C., Brewer, M., & Wieck, K. L. (2017). Using a Delphi method to identify human factors contributing to nursing errors. *Nursing Forum, 52*(3), 173–179.

Salar, A., Kiani, F., & Rezaee, N. (2020). Preventing the medication errors in hospitals: A qualitative study. *International Journal of Africa Nursing Sciences, 13.*

Thomas, L., Donohue-Porter, P., & Fishbein, J. (2017). Impact of interruptions, distractions, and cognitive load on procedure failures and medication administration errors. *Journal of Nursing Care Quality, 32*(4), 309-317.

Consequences of Nursing Errors

4

Nursing errors can be associated with a variety of patient outcomes. A near miss is when an error does not actually reach the patient but has the potential to cause harm. A near miss is an opportunity to identify a breakdown in the process before patient harm actually occurs (American Society for Healthcare Risk Management 2014; Maryniak 2018). One example of a near miss is a nurse who takes a vial of heparin out of the medication dispensary cabinet to flush a central line. The heparin flush should be a concentration of 10 units/mL. When the nurse double checks the vial, she sees the concentration is heparin 1000 units/mL. The nurse does not give the medication, and reports the incident to the pharmacy, as the medication drawer was stocked with the incorrect concentration of heparin.

No harm means that although an event reached a patient, there was no harm (American Society for Healthcare Risk Management 2014; Maryniak 2018). An illustration of an incident with no harm is a patient is to receive a dose of omeprazole before meals. The nurse brings in the patient's dose at 0900 and discovers that the patient ordered food and ate at 0700. This is an error because it was due prior to food, but there was no patient harm as a result of the error. The nurse then adjusts the time on the medication administration record for future doses, so that the omeprazole is given before the patient's meal.

© The Author(s), under exclusive license to Springer Nature Switzerland AG 2022
K. Maryniak, R. Garrett, *Preventing Errors and Pitfalls in Nursing with Infectious Patients*, https://doi.org/10.1007/978-3-030-86728-7_4

Mild harm includes minimal symptoms or injury with minor interventions, observation, or increased length of stay (American Society for Healthcare Risk Management 2014; Maryniak 2018). An instance of mild harm is a patient is given insulin based on a sliding scale. The last point of care blood glucose level was done by the nursing assistant over 90 min earlier. The nurse administers insulin based on this old glucose level. Within 15 min, the patient is diaphoretic with an altered level of consciousness. When the glucose level is rechecked, it is too low, and the patient requires oral glucose to bring his levels up. This is an error because the insulin should have been adjusted to what the patient's current blood glucose was. Interventions were needed to stabilize the patient, and there was increased monitoring needed. There was no lasting harm.

Moderate harm means that the patient has a bodily or psychological injury, which affects quality of life or function (American Society for Healthcare Risk Management 2014; Maryniak 2018). An example is a patient who is identified as a high fall risk in the emergency room. She is left on a gurney with the side rails up. The patient cannot reach her call bell and tries to call for assistance to the restroom. She gets up on her own and attempts to get out of bed. As a result, the patient falls and breaks her radius. This is moderate harm as there was a patient injury which affected the patient's quality of life. With a break in her arm, the harm is temporary until the bone heals.

Severe harm indicates physical or psychological injury to a patient, which significantly affects function or quality of life (American Society for Healthcare Risk Management 2014; Maryniak 2018). One case of severe harm is a patient who had extensive spinal surgery, including spinal fusion, with an expected stay in hospital for 3–5 days. Sequential compression devices (SCDs) were ordered, to be used when the patient was not ambulating. On day one, a nurse helped the patient ambulate to the restroom, and left the SCDs off the patient when she assisted him back to bed. In report, she told the oncoming nurse that the patient was ambulating. The SCDs were not replaced. On day four, the patient complained of pain in his right calf. It was discovered that he had developed a deep vein thrombosis (DVT). The patient needed an extended stay in the hospital to treat the DVT, and he went on to develop post-thrombotic syndrome. This was an error, as the SCDs should have been on as ordered. The harm was severe, with significant effects to the patient's quality of life.

Death is the last patient outcome as a result of an event (American Society for Healthcare Risk Management 2014; Maryniak 2018). One example is a patient who was ordered IV heparin via a weight-based protocol. The patient was weighed on admission by the nursing assistant, who entered the height and weight into the electronic record. The patient's weight was measured in pounds, and the height was reported by the patient in feet and inches. The nursing assistant then converted the measurements to metric to enter in the record. However, she transposed incorrectly. The height should have been 179 cm (5.9 ft.), and the patient's weight was 83 kg (182 pounds). What was entered into the record was 179 kg for weight, which is the equivalent of 394 pounds. When the heparin was ordered, the nurse entered the patient's recorded weight (179 kg) into the smart pump, which calculated the amount of heparin. The error was caught at shift change when the oncoming nurse noted the weight was incorrect by her assessment (the patient did not appear to be 394 pounds). At that time, the heparin was stopped and labs were ordered. The patient ended up with a cerebral bleed and died.

Errors related to the care, isolation, and precautions with infectious patients can not only harm the patient in the room but can possibly harm others. Failure to perform hand hygiene, use PPE inappropriately, or errors with PPE doffing can increase the risk of exposure to the healthcare professional through contamination. This in turn can put the caregiver at risk, as well as increased the risk of spreading infectious diseases to others. A higher chance of contagion spread to other patients or even loved ones of the healthcare professional at home may occur (Fan et al. 2020). Examples include the spread of MDROs in a hospital setting, such as MRSA in a neonatal intensive care unit (NICU). MRSA can often be spread by individuals who are colonized with the bacteria, usually from a community-acquired setting. Many studies have shown that outbreaks in a NICU setting can be traced to a healthcare professional who unknowingly passes along MRSA to these vulnerable patients (Brown et al. 2019; Huang et al. 2019; Popoola et al. 2014). Diligent hand hygiene and appropriate use of PPE can help prevent these outbreaks, along with other strategies.

Avoidable patient harm that can occur because of errors include morbidity and increased mortality. Both short-term and long-term effects may be seen. Hospital-acquired conditions such as CLABSIs, CAUTIs, VTE, VAEs, pressure injuries, and other hospital-acquired infections can cause unnecessary patient pain and suffering, complex conditions, potential disability, and impact on both physical and psychological states. Preventable falls in hospitals can also occur, contributing to the same issues. Other consequences include longer lengths of stay (and all of the risks inherent with that), as well as increased costs to the healthcare system (Panagioti et al. 2019).

A CLABSI is a central line-associated blood stream infection. The most vulnerable patients for developing CLABSIs are neonatal, pediatric, immunocompromised, and intensive care patients, due to the high utilization rates of central lines. CLABSI rates have been 4.1–5.3 cases per 1000 patient line days internationally (Agency for Healthcare Research and Quality 2020; Asia Pacific Society of Infection Control 2015). CLABSI is associated with high mortality and morbidity among the healthcare-acquired infections, due to bacteremia or fungal invasion, at a rate of 20,000–30,000 people each year (Agency for Healthcare Research and Quality [AHRQ] 2020; Asia Pacific Society of Infection Control 2015). Excess mortality examines additional deaths that are directly related to an infectious HAC. One meta-analysis that was done estimated that there are 150 excess deaths per 1000 cases of CLABSI, which is a rate of 0.15 (AHRQ 2017). Even in situations where there is no patient death, developing a CLABSI can cause the patient pain and anguish.

A CAUTI is a catheter-associated urinary tract infection. The most vulnerable patients for developing a CAUTI are geriatric, immunocompromised, and those with prolonged use of indwelling catheters. CAUTI rates are approximately 4.8 per 1000 catheter days internationally (Nicastri and Leone 2021). Approximately 19,000–20,000 cases of CAUTI are reported in the United States per year (U.S. Department of Health and Human Services 2021). However, it is estimated that 150 million people worldwide develop a CAUTI every year (Öztürk and Murt 2020). A meta-analysis that was done estimated that there are 36 excess deaths per 1000 cases of CAUTI, which is a rate of 0.036 (AHRQ 2017). Developing a CAUTI can be painful and create other patient complications.

Venous thromboembolism (VTE) includes development of a deep vein thrombosis (DVT) and/or a pulmonary embolism (PE). Patients at highest risk for developing VTE include those with extended hospital stays, surgical patients, decreased mobility, oncology patients, and those over the age of 60 (International Society on Thrombosis and Haemostasis [ISTH] 2022). A meta-analysis that was done estimated that there are 43 excess deaths per 1000 cases of VTE, which is a rate of 0.043 (AHRQ 2017). Worldwide, there are approximately ten million cases every year, with 60% percent of cases related to hospitalization. VTE is a leading cause of death and disability (ISTH 2022).

Ventilator-associated events (VAEs) are those that cause deterioration in respiratory status after a period of stability or improvement on the ventilator, with evidence of infection or inflammation, and laboratory evidence of respiratory infection. Ventilator-associated pneumonia (VAP) is one form of VAE, but other types are also included. VAP is a common hospital-acquired infection in intensive care units. International rates of VAE may be difficult to ascertain, as there are multiple factors regarding capturing and reporting incidents of VAE aside from VAP, with some ranges between 6 and 107 per 1000 ventilator days. One study estimates a rate of 23.72 cases of VAE for every 1000 ventilator days (He et al. 2021). For VAP alone, excess deaths are approximately 0.14, or 140 patients per 1000 cases (AHRQ 2017).

Pressure injuries are those that cause localized injury to the skin and underlying tissue. These injuries may or may not be pressure ulcers, and are generally seen over a bony prominence. Pressure injuries are caused by pressure and shear, or a combination of both. Vulnerable patients are those who have limited mobility, geriatric, immunocompromised, and have malnutrition. Prevalence of pressure injuries is approximately 12.8% of all hospitalized patients globally (Li et al. 2020). Excess mortality was estimated at 0.041, or 41 excess deaths for every 1000 pressure injury cases (AHRQ 2017).

Preventable falls are another concern in hospital, with an estimate of 3.56 falls per 1000 patient days globally. Of those patients that fall, 26–44% are injured as a result of the fall (Stephenson et al. 2016; Walsh et al. 2018). Patients at risk include those who are geriatric, pediatric, confused, impulsive, taking certain medications, those who experience difficulties with balance or have impaired mobility, and patients with a previous history of falls. Excess mortality was estimated at 0.05, or 50 excess deaths for every 1000 patient falls (AHRQ 2017).

Medication errors can also range in patient harm, from near misses to patient death. Medication errors may also cause adverse drug events (ADEs), which are often associated with patient harm. Errors associated with high-risk medications are those that often lead to severe harm, disability, or even death. Preventable patient injury from medication errors, although not common, can have a long-term impact on the patient and family (Afreen et al. 2021).

An ADE is a harm that occurs as a result of medication. Not all ADEs are result of an error. For example, heparin-induced thrombocytopenia (HIT) is a reaction that occurs from the use of heparin. HIT is considered an ADE, even when the medication is administered appropriately. A preventable ADE is one that is associated with a medication error which causes patient harm. It is estimated that about 5% of all hospitalized patients experience a preventable ADE (PSNet 2019). Risk factors for an ADE in hospital are geriatric patients, neonatal and pediatric patients, polypharmacy, high alert medications, use of look-alike sound-alike medications, and ineffective processes or noncompliance with safe medication administration (PSNet 2019). Excess mortality was estimated at 0.012, or 12 excess deaths for every 1000 ADEs (AHRQ 2017).

Nursing errors can also impact the organization itself. Patient harm resulting from errors has financial effects. There are higher costs associated with longer lengths of stay. And hospital-acquired conditions are not reimbursed by insurance companies. The additional costs for a patient who develops a CLABSI is an average of

$48,000 US dollars, with a range of $27,000–$69,000 (AHRQ 2017). For CAUTIs, it is estimated that the additional cost is over $13,000 per patient, with a range of $5000–$22,000 (AHRQ 2017). Estimated added costs for VTE is an average of $17,000, with a range of $12,000–$23,000; this does not include the costs associated with patient deaths (AHRQ 2017). VAE also has associated costs, at an average $47,000 for VAP, and a range of $22,000–$72,000 (AHRQ 2017). The additional average cost for a pressure injury is $14,500, with a range up to $41,000 (AHRQ 2017). Falls have an average added cost of $6694 per fall, with a range of $1300–$15,000 US dollars (AHRQ 2017). Additional costs for ADEs are estimated at $5800, ranging from $4000–$15,000 (AHRQ 2017).

Additionally, there may be lawsuits against an organization for patient harm that is caused by error. The lawsuits themselves can cost an organization financially, but the public perception of the organization may also be affected. Long-term, the organization's reputation may be affected, which can lead to further negative financial impact (Adler et al. 2018).

Errors that occur in healthcare can also have effects on others. Trust between the patient, family, and the healthcare team can be negatively affected by an error. This can occur even if there is disclosure about the error, although the impact on the patient's perception may be improved with disclosure. The Institute of Medicine's report, *To Err is Human* (2000), most errors are systemic but often decrease trust in the healthcare professional who made the error. Institutions that are not proactive, transparent, or create action when an error occurs can cause a patient to feel betrayed. This betrayal is often directed at the healthcare professional, rather than being at the organization that had systemic issues (Smith 2017).

The healthcare professional themselves may also be impacted by an error. Second victim syndrome is a term for a healthcare professional, such as a nurse, who has committed an error. The professional feels responsible, particularly if the error is associated with a poor outcome. The person may feel shame, guilt, anxiety, grief, depression, compassion dissatisfaction, burnout, secondary traumatic stress, and physical manifestations. The psy-

chological effects are not just about responsibility but goes deeper
to where the healthcare professional can be traumatized as a result
of the event (Ozeke et al. 2019).

References

Adler, L., Yi, D., Li, M., McBroom, B., Hauck, L., … & Classen, D. (2018).
    Impact of inpatient harms on hospital finances and patient clinical out-
    comes. *Journal of Patient Safety, 14*(2), 67-73.

Afreen, N., Padilla-Tolentino, E., & McGinnis, B. (2021). Identifying poten-
    tial high-risk medication errors using telepharmacy and a web-based sur-
    vey tool. *Innovations in Pharmacy, 12*(1), 10.

Agency for Healthcare Research and Quality (AHRQ). (2017). Estimating
    the additional hospital inpatient cost and mortality associated with
    selected hospital-acquired conditions. https://www.ahrq.gov/hai/pfp/
    haccost2017-results.html

Agency for Healthcare Research and Quality (AHRQ). (2020). Guide:
    Purpose and use of CLABSI tools. https://www.ahrq.gov/hai/clabsi-tools/
    guide.html

American Society for Healthcare Risk Management. (2014). Serious safety
    events: A focus on harm classification: Deviation in care as link. http://
    www.ashrm.org/pubs/files/white_papers/SSE-2_getting_to_zero-9-
    30-14.pdf

Asia Pacific Society of Infection Control. (2015). APSIC guide for prevention
    of central line associated bloodstream infections (CLABSI). https://apsic-
    apac.org/wp-content/uploads/2016/09/APSIC-CLABSI-guidelines-
    FINAL-20-Jan-2015.pdf

Brown, N., Reacher, M., Rice, W., Roddick, I., Reeve, L., … & Enoch, D.
    (2019). An outbreak of methicillin-resistant staphylococcus aureus colo-
    nization in a neonatal intensive care unit: use of a case-control study to
    investigate and control it and lessons learnt. *Journal of Hospital Infections,
    103*(1), 35-43.

Fan, J., Jiang, Y., Hu, K., Chen, X., Xu, Q., … & Liang, S. (2020). Barriers to
    using personal protective equipment by healthcare staff during the
    COVID-19 outbreak in China. *Medicine, 99*(48), e23310.

He, Q., Wang, W., Zhu, S., Wang, M., Kang, Y., … & Sun, X. (2021). The
    epidemiology and clinical outcomes of ventilator-associated events
    among 20,769 mechanically ventilated patients at intensive care units: An
    observational study. *Critical Care, 25*(44). https://ccforum.biomedcen-
    tral.com/articles/10.1186/s13054-021-03484-x#citeas

Huang, H., Ran, J., Yang, J., Li, P., Zhuang, G. (2019). Impact of MRSA
    transmission and infection in a neonatal intensive care unit in China: A

bundle intervention study during 2014-2017. *BioMed Research International,* 2019. https://www.hindawi.com/journals/bmri/2019/5490413/

Institute of Medicine. (2000) *To err is human: Building a safer health system.* National Academy Press.

International Society on Thrombosis and Haemostasis. (2022). Open your eyes to venous thromboembolism (VTE). https://www.worldthrombosis-day.org/issue/vte/

Li, Z, Lina, F., Thalibb, L., & Chaboyera, W. (2020). Global prevalence and incidence of pressure injuries in hospitalised adult patients: A systematic review and meta-analysis. *International Journal of Nursing Studies, 105.* https://www.sciencedirect.com/science/article/pii/S0020748920300316?via%3Dihub

Maryniak, K. (2018). *Medication errors: Best practices for prevention* (webinar). Lorman.

Nicastri, E., & Leone, S. (2021). Guide to infection control in the healthcare setting: Healthcare associated urinary tract infections. https://isid.org/guide/hospital/urinary-tract-infections/

Ozeke, O., Ozeke, V., Coskun, O., & Budakoglu, I. I. (2019). Second victims in health care: current perspectives. *Advances in Medical Education and Practice, 10,* 593–603.

Öztürk R, Murt A. (2020). Epidemiology of urological infections: A global burden. *World Journal of Urology, 38*(11), 2669-2679.

Panagioti, M., Khan, K., Keers, R., Abuzour, A., Phipps, D., … & Ashcroft, D. (2019). Prevalence, severity, and nature of preventable patient harm across medical care settings: Systematic review and meta-analysis *BMJ, 366,* l4185.

Popoola, V., Budd, A., Wittig, S., Ross, T., Aucott, S., … & Milstone, A. M. (2014). Methicillin-resistant staphylococcus aureus transmission and infections in a neonatal intensive care unit despite active surveillance cultures and decolonization: Challenges for infection prevention. *Infection Control and Hospital Epidemiology, 35*(4), 412–418.

PSNet. (2019). Medication errors and adverse drug events. https://psnet.ahrq.gov/primer/medication-errors-and-adverse-drug-events

Smith, C. (2017). First, do no harm: Institutional betrayal and trust in health care organizations. *Journal of Multidisciplinary Healthcare, 10,* 133-144.

Stephenson, M., Mcarthur, A., Giles, K., Lockwood, C., Aromataris, E., & Pearson, A. (2016). Prevention of falls in acute hospital settings: A multisite audit and best practice implementation project. *International Journal for Quality in Health Care, 28*(1), 92–98.

U.S. Department of Health and Human Services. (2021). Catheter-associated urinary tract infections. https://arpsp.cdc.gov/profile/infections/cauti?redirect=true

Walsh, C., Liang, L., Grogan, T., Coles, C., McNair, N., & Nuckols, T. (2018). Temporal trends in fall rates with the implementation of a multifaceted fall prevention program: Persistence pays off. *The Joint Commission Journal on Quality and Patient Safety, 44*(1), 75-83.

Monitoring for and Detecting Nursing Errors

Identifying errors can be difficult and time-consuming. Most hospitals have an event reporting system that is used to track and trend events once identified. Even more worrisome are the errors that go undetected or unreported due to fear of punishment. It is important for hospitals to adopt a safety program that is nonpunitive to encourage event reporting, a culture of open communication, transparency, and a quality assurance program that proactively monitors for abnormalities. Hospitals should have a strong internal audit program, including proactive risk assessments to help identify errors that may not be reported.

What do nurses spend the majority of their time doing? Sometimes we think that if we get them to document more the outcomes will be better. Documentation is *part* of a process and should not be used to control a process. Nothing is more frustrating to a nurse than overcomplicated documentation that takes their time away from the patient. Documentation should help guide the nurse but not be overly burdensome (Maryniak 2021). Nurses need to spend their critical thinking skills on the patient assessment and needs, not on remembering all the nuances of documentation requirements.

Documentation should direct the nurse in telling the patient story in a way that the next caregivers understand what they need to provide good care (Maryniak 2021). If nurses are struggling with documentation, it is probably a good idea to assess how the

© The Author(s), under exclusive license to Springer Nature
Switzerland AG 2022
K. Maryniak, R. Garrett, *Preventing Errors and Pitfalls in Nursing
with Infectious Patients*, https://doi.org/10.1007/978-3-030-86728-7_5

nursing documentation is set up. Ask this question: "Is our documentation set up in a way that helps guide the nurse to be successful and gives the appropriate information?" If there are a lot of documentation errors and/or handoff events, the documentation templates should probably be examined.

A root cause analysis (RCA) is a process of working towards discovering the real cause of a problem. The focus is on resolving the actual cause, rather than just looking at the symptoms of the issue. Contributing factors are identified during discussion of the event. An RCA does not need to be done with every problem, as it is a time-consuming process. However, there are times when an RCA is required, such as with serious safety events (e.g., never events, severe patient harm), repeat safety events, reportable patient injury (e.g., hospital-acquired infection, fall with injury), a near-miss with high potential for harm, based on patient or family complaints, and at the discretion of leadership.

One method of analysis for an RCA is where a team looks at five "whys." In this method, the question "why" is asked repeatedly until the original reason for the error, also known as the root cause of a problem, is found (Maryniak 2019). See also Fig. 5.1. A visual diagram, such as a fishbone, may be a useful tool to depict the contributing factors (see Fig. 5.2). Alternatively, the data about contributing factors from the RCA discussion can be listed in a table (see Fig. 5.3).

Many staff and leaders have been involved in root cause analysis or improvement plans. Following an RCA, a plan of corrective

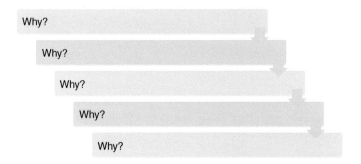

Fig. 5.1 Example of the "five whys"

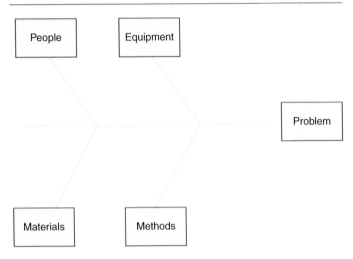

Fig. 5.2 Example of a fishbone diagram. Maryniak (2019). *Professional nursing practice in the United States: An overview for international nurses, and those along the continuum from new graduates to experienced nurses.* Author. (Used with permission)

Category	Contributing Factors
People	
Processes	
Equipment, supplies	
Culture	
Communication	
Staffing, training	

Fig. 5.3 Example of contributing factors table

action should be developed. These plans should include measurable and effective goals. An example of a table used for a corrective action is in Fig. 5.4. The key to making and sustaining actual improvement from an RCA is to determine goals and actions that are reasonable, actionable, and valuable.

What is the first thing that is suggested when there is an error? Education and some form of documentation audit. How is that working out? Did the investigation get to the root cause of the error? Who does the audits—the nurses that are telling everyone they have less time to spend with their patients? How can we help our nurses be successful in times of crisis and pandemics? We need to get back to the basics and look at our processes and workspaces. If we can get the waste out of our processes, we can help improve our outcomes. Waste can be time spent searching for supplies, over documentation, visual clutter, constant interruptions…the list goes on. Are there unnecessary steps in your processes that do not add value to the process? In Lean Six Sigma we use the term "value added" for process steps (Sweeney 2016). If a step does not add value, cannot be done right the first time, and is not something the customer (patient or regulatory agency) is willing to pay for then that step should be eliminated if possible.

If there are multiple errors found in a process that have different root causes, a good consideration would be to complete a Failure Modes and Effects Analysis (FMEA) to assess for vulnerability in the process. An FMEA can help identify vulnerable process steps, prioritize them by risk stratification, and implement mitigation strategies to decrease or eliminate the vulnerability (see also Fig. 5.5).

Corrective Action	Measure of Success	Responsible Party	Due to Review

Fig. 5.4 Corrective action planning table

Failure Modes and Effects Analysis (FMEA) Form

Product/Cell: Patient status assignment
Process: Admission
Problem: Delay in throughput/pt flow
Prepared By: Nurse Manager Jones

Severity (SEV) How severe is the effect on the customer? (5 = Most Severe, 1 = Least Severe)
Probability of Occurrence (OCC) How often does the cause or FM occur? (5 = Highest Occurrence, 1 = Lowest Occurrence)
Detectability (DET) How well can you detect the cause or FM using the current controls? (5 = Most Difficult to Detect, 1 = Easily Detected)
Risk Priority Number (RPN) What is the measure of process risk related to the effects, causes & controls? (RPN = SEV x OCC x DET)

Process Step/Input [What is the process step?]	Potential Failure Mode [What can go wrong with the process step/output (Ys)?]	Potential Failure Effects (What is the impact on the customer or internal requirements?)	S E V	Potential Causes [What are the root cause reasons (Xs) for the process step/output to go wrong?]	O C C	Current Controls [What are the existing controls that prevent or detect either the cause or the FM prior to leaving the process step?]	D E T	R P N	Actions Recommended [What are the actions for reducing the OCC of the cause or improving DET ?]	Plans / Responsibility [What is the target completion date and who is responsible?]	S E V	O C C	D E T	R P N
Admission through ED: orders written by physician	MD have 12 hours to complete orders	if pts condition changes - patient safety compromised	5	process allows	5	none	5	125	Hospitalists will see patient within 30 minutes arrival to floor.					0
	accepting MD not identified	patient safety compromised	5	MD availability/MD on call not clear for group	2	No admission of patient without orders (some slip through)	2	20						
	physician writes orders for bed placement before tests/results are reviewed	Inappropriate bed placement - patient safety compromised	4	lab/xray delay, high census, MD perception of high census to move pt faster	4	None	5	80	TBD by Throughput Committee					

Fig. 5.5 Example of an FMEA

A culture of transparency and open communication is important to increase safety and decrease errors. This does not just happen; it must be planned and groomed. Many organizations that adopt lean principles use a type of daily management system to ensure open communication between frontline staff and leadership. This can be as simple as a whiteboard used to communicate frontline needs and leadership expectations. Criteria is established to note the conditions for the shift, if there need to be adjustments to workflow due to call offs, number of patients in isolation, if there is equipment unavailable so staff are aware and do not have to spend unnecessary time looking for a piece of equipment that is not available, etc. Leaders can use the board to help guide their rounding and to alert staff to new processes or process changes. The purpose is to improve safety and quality of care for patients by ensuring that those who care for the patients are well equipped, those who lead the caregivers are well informed, and ensure a connection to purpose.

An example of a daily management board includes the following information:

- Census, number of patients in isolation.
- Staffing available for the shift and on call staff available.
- Supplies that are on backorder, broken or missing equipment, and estimated time available.
- Identification of high-risk patients including those with indwelling urinary catheters, high-risk skin breakdown, high fall risk, etc.
- New process, change in current process.

The caregivers can be better prepared for the shift and aware of the department issues. The leaders can use the information to prioritize their rounding and monitor high-risk patients in the department. Leaders can have a bigger impact on safety if they assist in real-time monitoring of high-risk patients and processes, instead of the status quo of retrospective monitoring. Real time, concurrent monitoring with immediate feedback is more effective in process control and connecting the purpose (the "why") than retrospective monitoring. If problems are found days, weeks, or months after the fact they are much harder to correct.

Using concurrent monitoring and mentoring can have an impact on the majority of healthcare-associated infections and accidents. It is known that with each day an indwelling urinary catheter is in place the chance of infection increases. Indwelling urinary catheters should only be used when clinically indicated and discontinued as soon as medically possible. Nurse-driven protocols for removal and tightly controlled use of devices can decrease infection rates substantially. Education should focus on the dangers of using devices when they are not medically necessary, and why it is important to remove these as soon as possible (Letica-Kriegel et al. 2019). The daily management board can alert nurses and leaders of the patients in the department with these devices to increase attention to care and removal of the devices. Charge nurses can assess if the device is medically necessary and the leader can assess that the care is appropriate, providing real-time feedback to caregivers present of any deviations noted. The old saying "it takes a village" applies to patient safety. It takes the entire team to keep patients safe. Tools such as a flowchart or value stream map can be useful to look at and evaluate the current state, and determine future state (see Figs. 5.6 and 5.7).

The only way a nurse leader can assess what their nurses are spending their time doing is by monitoring them where the work is happening. We call this in Lean Six Sigma going to the Gemba—going to where the work happens (Sweeney 2016). It is the responsibility of nursing leadership to provide the tools and resources the nurse needs to provide a high quality patient care. The only way to truly assess this is by going to where the work is being done and watching, asking questions, and seeing what works and what does not work.

An example of going to the Gemba was at a facility to help reduce medication errors in the behavior health department. When reviewing the events, it was noted that there was a high number of errors at a specific time of the day. Observations during that specific time of day, chosen to watch the medication pass, demonstrated that the nurse was interrupted more than 30 times during the medication pass. There was an immediate review of the medication records, and several missed doses and incorrectly administered doses of medications were found. This information was provided to the department director, and the location of the medication pass for this department was changed. This in turn lead to a decrease in medication errors by

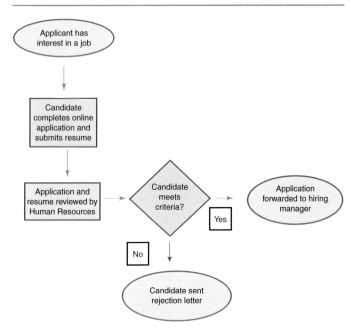

Fig. 5.6 Example of flowchart. Maryniak (2019). *Professional nursing practice in the United States: An overview for international nurses, and those along the continuum from new graduates to experienced nurses.* Author. (Used with permission)

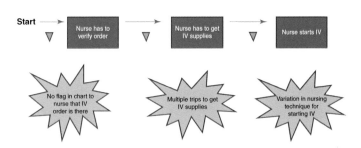

Fig. 5.7 Example of value stream analysis. Maryniak (2019). *Professional nursing practice in the United States: An overview for international nurses, and those along the continuum from new graduates to experienced nurses.* Author. (Used with permission)

over 50%. The nurses did not realize they were interrupted so often because they were so used to getting disrupted. This was eye-opening to the director and the nurses. Therefore, it is important for leaders to go where the work is and watch. The caregivers do not always recognize the contributing factors to errors because they develop a bias to them. Having fresh eyes on a situation can help find contributing factors that can be mitigated or even eliminated.

Standard work is also important to ensure that all caregivers complete processes the same and the outcomes are predictable. It would be very difficult to monitor a process if there is no standard way agreed on to complete the process. There are best practices available for many of the safety protocols, including monitoring and documentation. There should be standard expectations for care of high-risk patient types that can be monitored easily by leadership. An example of going back to indwelling urinary catheters includes monitoring the care bundle. The caregivers should be aware of the best practices caring for patients with indwelling urinary catheters, including avoiding dependent loops, keeping the bag below the bladder, securing the device so it does not pull, ensuring the bag is emptied appropriately, etc. This should be easy to understand and easy to monitor. If it is not written down, it is not standard work.

Another concept of lean principles is mutual respect. Leaders are responsible for leading by example, managing up their peers and staff in a way that builds mutual respect. This further improves the culture of safety in facilities that is imperative for patient safety and high quality of care. When a leader focuses on processes and does not blame caregivers immediately for errors, caregivers are more likely to report errors because they feel safe to do so. Transparency is a two-way street when it comes to safety and high reliability. If the leaders make promises, it should be transparent to the staff so they are held accountable for their actions as well.

You really do get what you plan for. Ask yourself the following:

- What is the communication plan from frontline caregivers to leaders, and vice versa?
- How are errors handled? Is the person to blame or does the organization look for the cause, contributing factors, and process issues?
- Do caregivers know what is expected of them?

- Are leaders' expectations clear with a connection to purpose?
- How does the organization identify high-risk patients in departments, and how does everyone work as a team to care for these patients and ensure they are not further compromised?
- Are the processes written in a way that all of the caregivers understand and follow them? If so, are they easy to find?
- Are there workarounds due to poor processes or obstacles that continue to cause barriers?

Other strategies to monitor for nursing errors include purposeful patient rounding (also known as hourly rounding) and leader rounding. Purposeful patient rounding is valuable for nursing staff to assess that patient needs are met while monitoring for patient safety. Rounding on patients by nursing leaders is also helpful to focus on patient safety. Examples include confirming fall precautions for those patients at risk, ensuring bundles are in compliance (such as central line bundles), and verifying indwelling urinary catheters are removed in a timely fashion (Maryniak 2019).

Bedside nurses are also essential in identifying potential and actual errors. Catching errors before they occur or recognizing areas of opportunity with policies, procedures, and protocols can make differences in current practices. With the increase in comorbidities and infections, it is important that nurses use tools to improve communication, transparency, and ensure the work is standardized and easily accessible and understood.

References

Letica-Kriegel, A. S., Salmasian, H., Vawdrey, D. K., Youngerman, B. E., Green, R. A., Furuya, E. Y., Calfee, D. P., & Perotte, R. (2019). Identifying the risk factors for catheter-associated urinary tract infections: a large cross-sectional study of six hospitals. *BMJ Open, 9*(2), e022137.

Maryniak, K. (2019). *Professional nursing practice in the United States: An overview for international nurses, and those along the continuum from new graduates to experienced nurses.* Author.

Maryniak, K. (2021). *Documentation for nurses* (4th ed.) (ebook). Elite Healthcare.

Sweeney, B. (2016). *Lean six sigma quickstart guide: The simplified beginner's guide to lean six sigma.* ClydeBank Media.

Best Practices to Prevent Nursing Errors

6

Scope of Practice

When looking at the potential for errors, nurses need to consider what is included in their nursing scope of practice. A scope of practice determines limitations and accountabilities of nurses. Although nursing scope of practice varies by location such as state or province of licensure, there are some general common considerations included within scope of practice. It is essential that nurses understand his or her scope of practice within their geographic location (e.g., state or province) (Maryniak 2018).

Examples of limitations within a nursing scope of practice are that a nurse can only administer medications that are ordered by a licensed provider; nurses cannot order medications. A provider may order protocols which identify specific circumstances and parameters for medication administration. Protocols may be implemented within an organization which define circumstances or parameters for medication administration. A common protocol is one created for hypoglycemia. In a hypoglycemia protocol, the parameters for blood glucose levels are described, and treatment is outlined. This may include administration of oral glucose, IV glucose, or glucagon as defined by blood glucose levels and patient response. It is also beyond the scope of the nurse to medically diagnose (Maryniak 2018).

© The Author(s), under exclusive license to Springer Nature Switzerland AG 2022
K. Maryniak, R. Garrett, *Preventing Errors and Pitfalls in Nursing with Infectious Patients*, https://doi.org/10.1007/978-3-030-86728-7_6

Nursing accountabilities within a scope of practice include that actions and interventions based on nursing assessment must either be ordered or included in policies, procedures, and protocols. This includes interventions that are part of medication administration. Nursing accountabilities include assessment, recognizing patient status changes, and using nursing judgment (Maryniak 2018).

Purposeful Patient Rounding

Purposeful patient rounding, formerly known as hourly rounding, is when nursing staff (nurses and nursing assistants) regularly go in to a patient's room during rounds. Previously, the reference to "hourly" rounding was focused more on the visit every hour. When viewed as this type of task, the intentional purpose behind rounding has been misidentified. There have been objective and subjective findings on the "drive-by," where nursing staff briefly look at the patient or ask "are you okay?". The purpose of effective rounding is to check frequently to assess safety and meet patient needs. Patient needs include if possessions and call bell within reach, and if the patient requires the use of the bathroom. The patient should also be asked what his or her pain level is, and if the patient needs to be repositioned. By meeting these needs, studies have shown improved patient safety and quality of care, reduction in patient falls and pressure injuries, decreased use of call lights, improved patient satisfaction scores, and enhanced nursing staff satisfaction (Ihediohanma 2020; Maryniak 2019).

Bedside Report

Bedside report, also known as shift report or nursing handoff, is another effective strategy to help prevent errors. With bedside report, both the oncoming and off-going nurses participate in handoff at the bedside of the patient. The goal is to include the patient and/or family in the report, which helps improve communication between staff and patients. Research has shown that communication breakdown is correlated with adverse events (AHRQ n.d.). Studies have also shown that bedside report increases patient satisfaction, and does improve nursing satisfaction as well, when it is done effectively (Dorvil 2018; Maryniak 2019). Standardized bedside report can focus on safety, such as double checks with patient lines and drains, activities, and plan of care. This interactive report can also assist in reinforcing patient and family teaching (AHRQ n.d.; Maryniak 2019).

A recommended process for bedside report is as follows:

- Introduce the nursing staff to the patient and family (if present), and invite them to participate in the bedside report.
- Access the health record.
- The off-going nurse will conduct a verbal report with the oncoming nurse, patient, and family (see standardized communication section below).
- Use words that the patient and family can understand.
- The oncoming nurse will conduct a safety inspection of the room, and a focused assessment of the patient.
    - Visually inspect all IV sites and tubing, wounds, incisions, drains, catheters, etc.
    - Visually sweep the room for any physical safety concerns.
- Both nurses will review tasks that were done, or need to be done, such as:
    - Labs or tests needed.
    - Medications administered.
- Identify the patient's and family's needs or concerns, and discuss their goal(s).
- Some questions to ask the patient and family may include:
    - "What could have gone better (during the shift)?"
    - "How is your pain right now?"
    - "Tell us how much you walked today."
    - "What concerns do you have?"
    - "What do you want to happen (during the next shift)?"
- Follow up to see if the goal was met during the next bedside report (AHRQ n.d.)

Standardized Communication

Standardized communication is essential in all aspects of healthcare. Effective communication between the interdisciplinary team and patients and families promote quality and safety. There are many formats for use in healthcare, whether it is for bedside report or discussing with other team members, such as a provider. The most common one used is the SBAR, which stands for **S**ituation, **B**ackground, **A**ssessment, and **R**ecommendations. An explanation of the SBAR components are:

- Situation: This is a brief description of what is happening with the patient. This should include the current assessment and vital signs.
- Background: This includes the pertinent history of this patient, as it relates to the problem. This may contain diagnosis, medications, laboratory values, and interventions.
- Assessment: This is the assessment of the situation. Describe what the problem is at this time.
- Recommendations: This is any specific request about what the patient needs. Or, during report, this component may be the recommendation of what the patient needs (AHRQ n.d.).

Another useful tool for standardized communication is the I-PASS, which stands for **I**llness severity, **P**atient summary, **A**ction list, **S**ituation awareness, and **S**ynthesis by receiver. Components of the I-PASS are:

- Illness severity: This is a description of how ill the patient is. This may also include code status.
- Patient summary: This is a brief patient overview, including pertinent information such as allergies, weight, hospital course, systems review (if concerns), any pertinent history.
- Action list: This includes tasks that are pending, such as laboratory results, procedures, and medications.
- Situation awareness: This gives specific information about interventions or what may potentially go wrong. This will help the other person anticipate problems, and be prepared.

- Synthesis by receiver: This allows for questions and clarifications, to ensure that information was received and understood (Blazin et al. 2020).

Strategies Specific to Infectious Patients

When working with infectious patients, nurses should be aware of the strategies to prevent contamination. This includes avoiding touching hands to face, and limiting touch of potentially contaminated surfaces. Standard precautions should be used judiciously with all patients, regardless of the level of isolation required (CDC 2017). Hand hygiene should be performed frequently and efficiently. Times identified when hand hygiene should be performed include before entering a patient room, before touching a patient, prior to any aseptic procedures, after exposure to blood or body fluids, following touching a patient, after touching the patient environment, and after leaving the patient room. Gloves should also be replaced when heavily soiled or torn (CDC n.d.). A commonly associated contributing cause to outbreaks of hospital-associated infections such as C. diff or MDROs is carrying organisms by the hands of nurses and other healthcare professionals (CDC 2019).

Steps for hand washing are:

1. Wet hands with clean, running water (warm or cold), turn off the tap, and apply soap.
2. Lather hands by rubbing them together with the soap. Lather the backs of the hands, between the fingers, and under the nails.
3. Scrub hands for at least 20 s. Need a timer? Hum the "Happy Birthday" song from beginning to end twice.
4. Rinse hands well under clean, running water.
5. Dry hands using a clean towel or air dry them (see Fig. 6.1).

Steps for hand hygiene using alcohol-based hand rub (ABHR) are:

1. Apply the gel product to the palm of one hand (read the label to learn the correct amount).

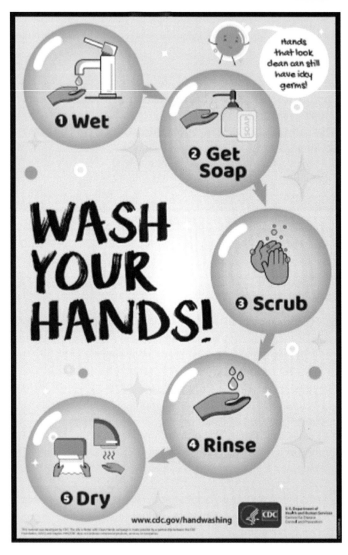

Fig. 6.1 Hand washing graphic. Materials developed by CDC. https://www.cdc.gov/handwashing/pdf/wash-your-hands-poster-english2020-p.pdf.   Reference to specific commercial products, manufacturers, companies, or trademarks does not constitute its endorsement or recommendation by the US Government, Department of Health and Human Services, or Centers for Disease Control and Prevention

2. Rub hands together.
3. Rub the gel over all the surfaces of hands and fingers until hands are dry. This should take around 20 s (see Fig. 6.2).

Understanding the PPE requirements for isolation and associated precautions is crucial. This includes communication and appropriate use of PPE in all areas of healthcare. Transporting patients who are in airborne precautions, for example, requires the use of a surgical mask with the patient, and either an N95 or PAPR for the staff interacting with the patient (CDC 2019).

It is important for nurses to understand the appropriate techniques for donning and doffing PPE, as this is a risk for both patients and the nurses themselves. For donning, the proper sequence of placing PPE is as follows:

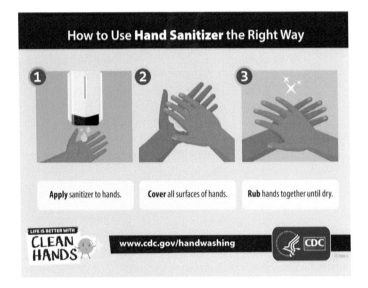

Fig. 6.2 Hand hygiene with ABHR graphic. Materials developed by CDC. https://www.cdc.gov/handwashing/pdf/326806-A_Hand-Sanitizer-SignageSticker-Update-final2_11x8.5in_printonly.pdf. Reference to specific commercial products, manufacturers, companies, or trademarks does not constitute its endorsement or recommendation by the US Government, Department of Health and Human Services, or Centers for Disease Control and Prevention

1. Gown—the gown should cover the full torso, neck to knees, arms to wrists. The gown should wrap around and be fastened at the neck and back.
2. Mask or respirator—secure ties at the back of the head and neck, fit the noseband to the bridge of the nose, fit the mask snug to the face and below the chin, and fit-check the respirator.
3. Eye protection—place safety goggles or face shield and adjust the fit.
4. Gloves—gloves should cover the wrists of the isolation gown. See also Fig. 6.3 (CDC n.d.).

For doffing PPE, there are two sequences that can be done to remove PPE. All PPE except a respirator should be removed prior to leaving a patient's room. The first order is:

1. Gloves—remember that the outside of the gloves are contaminated; if there is touch of the outside of the glove hand hygiene should be immediately performed. Using one glove, grab the palm of the other glove and pull off, holding the used glove in the hand still gloved. The ungloved hand should slide under the other glove, peeling the glove over the second glove. Dispose gloves in a garbage container.
2. Eye protection—remember that the outside of the eye protection is contaminated; if there is touch of the outside then hand hygiene should be immediately performed. Remove goggles or face shield by the back, either at the band or earpieces. If reusable, place in the designated container. If disposable, place eye protection in a garbage container.
3. Gown—remember that the front and gown sleeves are contaminated; if there is touch of those areas then hand hygiene should be immediately performed. Undo the gown ties and remove the gown by grabbing the inside of the gown only and pulling away from neck and shoulders. Turn the gown inside out, fold or roll it into a bundle, and dispose in a garbage container.
4. Mask or respirator—remember that the outside of the mask or respirator is contaminated; if there is a touch then hand hygiene should be immediately performed. Remove bottom ties or

SEQUENCE FOR PUTTING ON PERSONAL PROTECTIVE EQUIPMENT (PPE)

The type of PPE used will vary based on the level of precautions required, such as standard and contact, droplet or airborne infection isolation precautions. The procedure for putting on and removing PPE should be tailored to the specific type of PPE.

1. GOWN

- Fully cover torso from neck to knees, arms to end of wrists, and wrap around the back
- Fasten in back of neck and waist

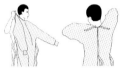

2. MASK OR RESPIRATOR

- Secure ties or elastic bands at middle of head and neck
- Fit flexible band to nose bridge
- Fit snug to face and below chin
- Fit-check respirator

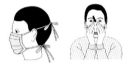

3. GOGGLES OR FACE SHIELD

- Place over face and eyes and adjust to fit

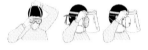

4. GLOVES

- Extend to cover wrist of isolation gown

USE SAFE WORK PRACTICES TO PROTECT YOURSELF AND LIMIT THE SPREAD OF CONTAMINATION

- Keep hands away from face
- Limit surfaces touched
- Change gloves when torn or heavily contaminated
- Perform hand hygiene

Fig. 6.3 PPE donning sequence. Materials developed by CDC. https://www.cdc.gov/hai/pdfs/ppe/ppe-sequence.pdf Reference to specific commercial products, manufacturers, companies, or trademarks does not constitute its endorsement or recommendation by the US Government, Department of Health and Human Services, or Centers for Disease Control and Prevention

bands first followed by those at the top, and discard them in a garbage container.

5. Hand hygiene should be performed immediately after PPE removal, either through handwashing or use of alcohol-based sanitizer. See also Fig. 6.4 (CDC n.d.)

The second possible sequence for appropriate doffing of PPE is:

1. Gown and gloves together—remember the front of the gown, sleeves, and outside of gloves are contaminated; if there is touch of those areas then hand hygiene should be immediately performed. Grab the front of the gown with gloved hands and pull away from the body so that the ties break. Turn the gown inside out, fold or roll it into a bundle, peeling off the gloves at the same times. Touch only the inside of the gown and gloves with bare hands. Place both gown and gloves into a garbage container.

2. Eye protection—remember that the outside of the eye protection is contaminated; if there is a touch of the outside then hand hygiene should be immediately performed. Remove goggles or face shield by the back, either at the band or earpieces. If reusable, place it in the designated container. If disposable, place eye protection in a garbage container.

3. Mask or respirator—remember that the outside of the mask or respirator is contaminated; if there is a touch then hand hygiene should be immediately performed. Remove bottom ties or bands first followed by those at the top, and discard them in a garbage container.

4. Hand hygiene should be performed immediately after PPE removal, either through handwashing or use of alcohol-based sanitizer. See also Fig. 6.5 (CDC n.d.)

When wearing an N95 mask, it is important to wear the appropriate size and have an effective seal. Fit testing of healthcare employees to determine the proper mask size should be done on a regular basis. Considerations for N95 masks are:

HOW TO SAFELY REMOVE PERSONAL PROTECTIVE EQUIPMENT (PPE) EXAMPLE 1

There are a variety of ways to safely remove PPE without contaminating your clothing, skin, or mucous membranes with potentially infectious materials. Here is one example. **Remove all PPE before exiting the patient room** except a respirator, if worn. Remove the respirator **after** leaving the patient room and closing the door. Remove PPE in the following sequence:

1. GLOVES

- Outside of gloves are contaminated!
- If your hands get contaminated during glove removal, immediately wash your hands or use an alcohol-based hand sanitizer
- Using a gloved hand, grasp the palm area of the other gloved hand and peel off first glove
- Hold removed glove in gloved hand
- Slide fingers of ungloved hand under remaining glove at wrist and peel off second glove over first glove
- Discard gloves in a waste container

2. GOGGLES OR FACE SHIELD

- Outside of goggles or face shield are contaminated!
- If your hands get contaminated during goggle or face shield removal, immediately wash your hands or use an alcohol-based hand sanitizer
- Remove goggles or face shield from the back by lifting head band or ear pieces
- If the item is reusable, place in designated receptacle for reprocessing. Otherwise, discard in a waste container

3. GOWN

- Gown front and sleeves are contaminated!
- If your hands get contaminated during gown removal, immediately wash your hands or use an alcohol-based hand sanitizer
- Unfasten gown ties, taking care that sleeves don't contact your body when reaching for ties
- Pull gown away from neck and shoulders, touching inside of gown only
- Turn gown inside out
- Fold or roll into a bundle and discard in a waste container

4. MASK OR RESPIRATOR

- Front of mask/respirator is contaminated — DO NOT TOUCH!
- If your hands get contaminated during mask/respirator removal, immediately wash your hands or use an alcohol-based hand sanitizer
- Grasp bottom ties or elastics of the mask/respirator, then the ones at the top, and remove without touching the front
- Discard in a waste container

5. WASH HANDS OR USE AN ALCOHOL-BASED HAND SANITIZER IMMEDIATELY AFTER REMOVING ALL PPE
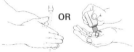

PERFORM HAND HYGIENE BETWEEN STEPS IF HANDS BECOME CONTAMINATED AND IMMEDIATELY AFTER REMOVING ALL PPE

CDC

Fig. 6.4 PPE doffing, sequence #1. Materials developed by CDC. https://www.cdc.gov/hai/pdfs/ppe/ppe-sequence.pdf Reference to specific commercial products, manufacturers, companies, or trademarks does not constitute its endorsement or recommendation by the US Government, Department of Health and Human Services, or Centers for Disease Control and Prevention

HOW TO SAFELY REMOVE PERSONAL PROTECTIVE EQUIPMENT (PPE) EXAMPLE 2

Here is another way to safely remove PPE without contaminating your clothing, skin, or mucous membranes with potentially infectious materials. **Remove all PPE before exiting the patient room** except a respirator, if worn. Remove the respirator **after** leaving the patient room and closing the door. Remove PPE in the following sequence:

1. GOWN AND GLOVES

- Gown front and sleeves and the outside of gloves are contaminated!
- If your hands get contaminated during gown or glove removal, immediately wash your hands or use an alcohol-based hand sanitizer
- Grasp the gown in the front and pull away from your body so that the ties break, touching outside of gown only with gloved hands
- While removing the gown, fold or roll the gown inside-out into a bundle
- As you are removing the gown, peel off your gloves at the same time, only touching the inside of the gloves and gown with your bare hands. Place the gown and gloves into a waste container

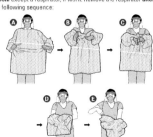

2. GOGGLES OR FACE SHIELD

- Outside of goggles or face shield are contaminated!
- If your hands get contaminated during goggle or face shield removal, immediately wash your hands or use an alcohol-based hand sanitizer
- Remove goggles or face shield from the back by lifting head band and without touching the front of the goggles or face shield
- If the item is reusable, place in designated receptacle for reprocessing. Otherwise, discard in a waste container

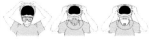

3. MASK OR RESPIRATOR

- Front of mask/respirator is contaminated — DO NOT TOUCH!
- If your hands get contaminated during mask/respirator removal, immediately wash your hands or use an alcohol-based hand sanitizer
- Grasp bottom ties or elastics of the mask/respirator, then the ones at the top, and remove without touching the front
- Discard in a waste container

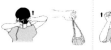

4. WASH HANDS OR USE AN ALCOHOL-BASED HAND SANITIZER IMMEDIATELY AFTER REMOVING ALL PPE

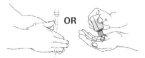

PERFORM HAND HYGIENE BETWEEN STEPS IF HANDS BECOME CONTAMINATED AND IMMEDIATELY AFTER REMOVING ALL PPE

Fig. 6.5 PPE doffing, sequence #2. Materials developed by CDC. https://www.cdc.gov/hai/pdfs/ppe/ppe-sequence.pdf Reference to specific commercial products, manufacturers, companies, or trademarks does not constitute its endorsement or recommendation by the US Government, Department of Health and Human Services, or Centers for Disease Control and Prevention

1. Place the N95 over the nose and under your chin. If the respirator has two straps, place one strap below the ears and one strap above.
2. If the N95 has a nose clip, the fingertips from both hands are used to mold the nose clip firmly against the nose and face. Do not pinch with one hand.
3. A seal check should be done every time an N95 is donned, and before entering a patient room.
4. Facial hair will cause the N95 to leak, so users should be clean-shaven; some types of facial hair are acceptable as long as it does not lie along the sealing area of the N95.
5. While wearing, if someone becomes dizzy, lightheaded, or nauseated, they leave the patient room, remove the N95, and get medical attention.
6. N95s should be discarded when it is increasingly difficult to breathe through, it becomes soiled, or if it is damaged.
7. Never touch the front of the N95 mask, as it may be contaminated.
8. Keep the N95 mask clean and dry, and follow the manufacturer's recommendations on use and storage. See also Fig. 6.6. (CDC 2020)

Errors related to violations, mistakes, and slips can be based on knowledge deficits (including misperception of risk) or poor time management. Knowing violations from reckless behaviors require accountability on behalf of the violator, as the behavior has a high risk of continuing. Equipment and environmental factors may also contribute to causing mistakes. These should be identified and addressed. Because slips are those errors associated with automatic behaviors, they are difficult to address. Focusing communications on awareness of unintentional behaviors, such as touching items or face with contaminated gloves, may be helpful. Evaluating the completeness and feasibility of policies, including reinforcing education are other strategies to assist in decreasing errors with PPE doffing and donning (Krein et al. 2018).

Important factors that contribute to healthcare-associated infections, such as C. diff, are environmental contamination and persistence of organisms (like spores) for extended periods of

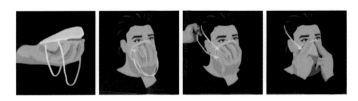

Fig. 6.6   N95 donning. Materials developed by CDC. https://blogs.cdc.gov/niosh-science-blog/2020/03/16/n95-preparedness/. Reference to specific commercial products, manufacturers, companies, or trademarks does not constitute its endorsement or recommendation by the US Government, Department of Health and Human Services, or Centers for Disease Control and Prevention

time. Use of appropriate products for disinfecting surfaces is vital, such as those that can kill spores associated with C. diff. Antibiotic and antimicrobial stewardship is also important to decrease the risk of developing MDROs or C. diff.

Approaches for Preventing CLABSIs

The best evidence for preventing CLABSIs include the use of bundles for both insertion and maintenance of central lines. For insertion, strategies include choosing the most appropriate insertion site based on the patient. The femoral site is not recommended, particularly with obese patients. Hand hygiene and aseptic technique adherence is important prior to insertion. Maximal sterile barriers are required for line insertion. The central line insertion site should be prepared with greater than 0.5% chlorhexidine and alcohol solution. Use of a chlorhexidine impregnated dressing is recommended for patients over the age of 18 (Association for Professionals in Infection Control and Epidemiology [APIC] 2015).

Effective hand hygiene and aseptic technique is also required for central line maintenance. Patients (over 2 months of age) should be bathed daily with a chlorhexidine solution. Prior to accessing a port of the central line, vigorous scrubbing with chlorhexidine, iodine, or 70% alcohol is needed. Access to devices is through sterile devices only. Gauze dressings should be changed at least every 48 h, and semipermeable dressings ought to be changed every 7 days. Dressings should also be immediately changed when soiled or loose. IV continuous administration sets should not be changed more frequently than every 96 h, and at least every 7 days. Tubing for blood, blood products, or lipid administration requires changing every 24 h. With administration of propofol, the tubing needs changing every 6–12 h or with a change in the vial. The need for continuing a central line is to be assessed daily, and lines should be immediately removed when no longer required (APIC 2015).

Best Practices for Avoiding CAUTIs

CAUTIs can occur with prolonged use of an indwelling urinary catheter, particularly with at-risk patients such as elderly, immunocompromised, or female. Use of a CAUTI prevention bundle can be effective in reducing the risk. The most effective strategy is to avoid insertion of an indwelling catheter unless absolutely necessary and removing them as soon as possible. Indications for indwelling catheters may be for urinary retention (if a bladder protocol is not effective), as required by a urologist, or comfort care. Use of indwelling catheters for surgery should be limited and removed as soon as able postoperatively. Patients in intensive care units do not require routine use of indwelling catheters (Saint et al. 2016).

Hand hygiene and aseptic technique is vital during catheter insertion and during catheter care. It is recommended to use closed, preconnected catheter systems. Other strategies as part of a bundle include assessing and avoiding kinking of the catheter and tubing, ensuring the collection bag is below the level of the bladder, and confirming the bag is not on the floor. Regular cleansing of the catheter and perineum is also needed. Ongoing assessment of the catheter and determination for ongoing use is also essential. Many organizations have a policy for use of a nurse-driven catheter removal protocol which, if used appropriately, can remove the catheter in a timelier fashion (Saint et al. 2016).

Strategies for Prevention of VTEs

Prevention strategies are essential for both deep vein thrombosis (DVT) and pulmonary embolism (PE), which encompass VTE. Hospitalized patients are at high risk for developing VTE based on time spent in bed, procedures or surgery, and disease processes which lead to hospitalization. Patients in hospital, with the exception of those on comfort care, require some form of VTE prophylaxis. This may include ambulation and the use of sequential compression devices (SCDs). Ambulation requirements are more significant than a patient just ambulating to the restroom. Studies recommend 275–900 steps per day, which is associated with better clinical outcomes (Jeong et al. 2020). SCDs must be on and functioning when the patient is in bed. Pharmacological prophylaxis, such as heparin or warfarin, may also be indicated. Patient and family education regarding the need for VTE prophylaxis is important to assist with compliance (Maryniak 2021).

Preventing Ventilator-Associated Events

Ventilator-associated events (VAEs) include ventilator-associated pneumonia (VAP), pulmonary edema, acute respiratory distress syndrome (ARDS), pulmonary embolism, and atelectasis. The longer a patient is on a mechanical ventilator, the higher the risk for developing VAEs. VAP is an infection within the airway following 48 h of intubation and is correlated with high mortality rates. Patients at high risk include the elderly, immunocompromised, and patients with preexisting respiratory illness or dysfunction (Klompas 2019).

Ventilator bundles are designed to prevent VAP, but the main initiative against preventing any VAE is to minimize the time the patient is on the ventilator. Strategies include using alternatives to intubation, assessing the need for ventilation daily, and weaning off the ventilator as soon as possible. Weaning from sedation is also important, and the use of spontaneous awakening with breathing trials is indicated. Other strategies include providing good oral care frequently with an antiseptic solution. Maintaining the head of the bed at 30–45° can prevent aspiration. Use of low tidal volumes and conservative fluid management are also good approaches (Klompas 2019).

Strategies for Preventing Pressure Injuries

Pressure injuries, also known as bedsores, pressure ulcers, or decubitus ulcers, are damage that occurs to the skin and soft tissues. Prolonged pressure, friction, shear, and poor nutritional status can predispose patients to develop pressure injuries. Pressure injuries may or may not be associated with pain. Hospitalized patients are at risk for pressure injuries due to disease processes, compromised circulation, procedures and surgery, prolonged sitting or time in bed, incontinence, medical devices, and pressure on bony prominences (Haesler 2019).

Performing comprehensive skin assessments is essential to identify patients at risk for pressure injury, and implementing individualized prevention plans. Standardized risk assessment tools should be used. It is recommended for two nurses to perform a comprehensive skin assessment on admission and following a transfer. Skin assessments using the appropriate tool should be performed at least daily and on discharge. The entire skin from head to toe should be examined for abnormalities. This requires visualization under clothes or gown, with particular focus on skin folds, body prominences, and under medical devices (Haesler 2019).

The skin should be compared symmetrically, noting any differences in skin color, temperature, or areas that do not blanch. Moisture, skin turgor, and skin integrity should be assessed. If wounds or discoloration is noted, this should be documented and photographed (Maryniak 2021).

Fall Prevention Approaches

Falls are defined as unplanned descent to the floor. In the United States alone, approximately 700,000–1,000,000 patients fall in healthcare settings each year, with 250,000 suffering from injury

(LeLaurin and Shorr 2019). Injuries associated with falls may range from bruises, lacerations, and fractures to internal bleeding and death. Patient assessment is a priority to identify patients at risk of falling and implementing individualized strategies to help prevent falls. Use of a standardized fall assessment tool is needed, which identifies risk factors for falling. Examples of risk factors include age, difficulty ambulating or transferring, frequent toileting needs, history of previous falls, medications, sensory impairment, alterations in mental status, and medical conditions (LeLaurin and Shorr 2019).

All patients should have standard fall precautions, such as orienting the patient to the room environment and call light, ensuring personal items and call light are within reach, and placing hospital beds in the lowest position while the patient is in bed. Brakes should be on hospital beds, chairs, and wheelchairs when stationary. Nonslip well-fitted footwear, such as socks, should be provided to patients. Appropriate lighting, including the use of night lights, and sturdy handrails in rooms, bathrooms, and halls are needed. Environments should be clean and clutter-free, with clean, dry floors. Safe patient handling techniques are essential when assisting patients, including the use of a gait belt when ambulating patients. Purposeful rounding on a regular basis, as aforementioned, can also assist in meeting patient needs and assessing safety, including measures for fall prevention (LeLaurin and Shorr 2019; Maryniak 2019).

Additional safety precautions are required for patients at risk for falls. These should be individualized to the patient. Interventions for risk factors should be implemented, such as supervising and reorienting patients with cognitive impairment, assessing medication effects, and creating a safe environment. Patients at high risk, particularly those with cognitive impairment and impulsivity, may require the use of a sitter to constantly monitor patient activity. The use of tele sitters is an alternative, but this is not recommended for patients who have altered mental status or cognitive impairment. Medication effects should be assessed by nurses, pharmacists, and providers to determine if there are alternatives which may decrease fall risk. Monitoring of patient vital signs and slow transitions to ambulating is essential if patient medication increases fall risk. Impairment in mobility may require the use of assistive devices, which should be easily accessible. Use of transfer devices or lifts may be necessary for safe patient handling (LeLaurin and Shorr 2019).

Education of patient and family, including the use of signs to remind them to ask for assistance with ambulating may be effective. Bed and chair alarms may also remind the patient to wait for help, but they are not an effective strategy for impulsive patients. Many times, the alarm may not be heard by staff until the patient is already out of the bed or chair (LeLaurin and Shorr 2019).

Many organizations have fall prevention programs which include the use of visual cues for the interdisciplinary team. Use of colored signs, socks, and wristbands can alert all team members that a patient is a fall risk (LeLaurin and Shorr 2019).

Best Practices Associated with Restraints

The use of restraints or seclusion is only for protecting the immediate physical safety of the patient or others. There must be an appropriate justification of the use of restraints or seclusion in which a provider order is needed, and this must be discontinued as soon as possible. Alternatives to restraints and seclusion must be used prior to implementation, based on a comprehensive assessment. If it is determined that restraint or seclusion is needed, then the least restrictive method must be used (CMS 2020).

Physical restraints include holding a patient down, use of all four side rails up (to prevent them from getting out of bed), net enclosure beds, limb restraints, vest restraints, and mittens if they are tied down or restricted the ability of the patient to use their hands. Chemical restraints involve the use of medications to control a patient's behavior. Seclusion is when the patient is involuntarily confined to an area, which is only allowed for the management of violent behavior (CMS 2020).

An order for restraints or seclusion is required from a provider. In the United States, there are time limits for orders. According to CMS (2020), for adults (18 years and older), the maximum is 4 h; for children and adolescents (9–17 years old), the maximum is

2 h; and for children (under 9 years old), the maximum is 1 h. After 24 h, the provider must see and assess the patient before writing further restraint or seclusion orders.

While using restraint or seclusion, the patient's condition must be monitored by a trained healthcare professional, including a nurse. The condition includes the patient's reaction and need to continue the intervention. If restraints are used, the patient's circulation and movement should be assessed (CMS 2020).

Strategies for Preventing Medication Errors

When looking at strategies to prevent medication errors, there are those at a system level to consider. The National Patient Safety Goals, developed by the Joint Commission, are used as standards for patient safety at organizations throughout the US. The goals are developed around areas that can be problems in healthcare and are a focus on safety. The 2022 goals include categories of patient identification and to use medicines safely. Other categories are focused on improving interdisciplinary clinical communication, reducing patient harm associated with clinical alarms, reducing risks of hospital-acquired infections, and identifying patient safety risks (The Joint Commission 2021b).

There are multiple strategies at the system level to help decrease the chance of medication errors, which should be incorporated into organizational processes. The use of two patient identifiers, such as name and date of birth, must be used with medication administration. All medications should be labeled, such as those in syringes or other containers. Anticoagulants, such as blood thinners, put patients at higher risk for complications. Extra care and assessment should be done with these patients. Maintaining medication reconciliation is important throughout the patient's continuum, including transition from hospital to home, and with every outpatient visit (Maryniak 2018).

Another important focus for system improvement is policies and procedures, such as those involving medication administration. These should be developed based on evidence and must meet regulatory and accreditation standards. Multidisciplinary team members provide key stakeholders who are involved in medication administration. Shared governance is effective by adding frontline staff who can add valuable insight into policies. Staff buy-in is also improved when they are part of the process, including policy development. Policies are those that must be followed, which differ from guidelines. Education about policies includes this fact, and staff need to be held accountable for following policies. Organizations need to clearly define reporting processes for medication errors. This may include verbal reporting, such as to a provider, and written or electronic reporting processes. Policies for security and access regarding medications should also be created for facilities. This includes those requirements for secured location of medication, and which employees are able to access medications (such as licensed personnel). Medication administration policies may also include use of technology such as barcoded medication administration, computerized provider order entry, and smart IV pumps (Maryniak 2018).

Other policy and procedure considerations include safety standards. Organizations should define unacceptable abbreviations. The Joint Commission (2021a) has a list of unacceptable abbreviations, and the Institute for Safe Medication Practices (ISMP) also has extended list of abbreviations, symbols, and other written information which can potentially cause medical errors (ISMP 2021). Unacceptable abbreviations must be defined within a facility. Reference lists are available through the Joint Commission and the Institute for Safe Medication Practices. Examples of unacceptable abbreviations include:

- Avoiding "u" and spelling out "units".
- Avoiding "IU" and spelling out "international units".
- Writing out "daily" and "every other day" rather than using "qd", and "qod".
- Not using trailing 0 after a decimal point.
- Using 0 before a decimal point.
- Writing out morphine sulfate or magnesium sulfate rather than abbreviating with "ms".
- Using "mL" rather than cc.
- Writing out "discharge" or "discontinue" rather than "d/c" abbreviation (ISMP 2021; The Joint Commission 2021a).

High-risk medications need to be defined within the organization as well. Practices related to high-risk medication also need to be documented. Strategies to decrease the risk of medication errors with high-risk medications (ISMP 2018) include:

- Standardization of ordering, storage, preparation, and administration of these medications.
- Improved access to information about these drugs.
- Access to high-alert medications should be limited.
- Supplementary labels and automated alerts can be used.
- Use of redundancies, such as independent double checks.

The ISMP (2018) also has a list of recommended high-risk medications, identified as those which can cause significant patient harm. These include classes of:

- adrenergic agonists, IV (e.g., epinephrine, phenylephrine, norepinephrine),
- adrenergic antagonists, IV (e.g., propranolol, metoprolol, labetalol),
- anesthetic agents, general, inhaled and IV (e.g., propofol, ketamine),
- antiarrhythmics, IV (e.g., lidocaine, amiodarone),
- antithrombotic agents, including anticoagulants (e.g., warfarin, low molecular weight heparin, unfractionated heparin); direct oral anticoagulants and factor Xa inhibitors (e.g., dabigatran, rivaroxaban, apixaban, edoxaban, betrixaban, fondaparinux); direct thrombin inhibitors (e.g., argatroban, bivalirudin, dabigatran); glycoprotein IIb/IIIa inhibitors (e.g., eptifibatide); thrombolytics (e.g., alteplase, reteplase, tenecteplase),
- cardioplegic solutions,
- chemotherapeutic agents, both parenteral and oral,
- dextrose, hypertonic, 20% or greater,
- dialysis solutions, both peritoneal and hemodialysis,
- epidural and intrathecal medications,
- inotropic medications, IV (e.g., digoxin, milrinone),

- insulin, subcutaneous and IV,
- liposomal forms of drugs (e.g., liposomal amphotericin B) and conventional counterparts (e.g., amphotericin B desoxycholate),
- moderate sedation agents, IV (e.g., dexmedetomidine, midazolam, lorazepam),
- moderate and minimal sedation agents, oral, for children (e.g., chloral hydrate, midazolam, ketamine [using the parenteral form]),
- opioids, including IV; oral (including liquid concentrates, immediate- and sustained-released formulations); transdermal,
- neuromuscular blocking agents (e.g., succinylcholine, rocuronium, vecuronium),
- parenteral nutrition preparations,
- sodium chloride for injection, hypertonic, greater than 0.9% concentration,
- sterile water for injection, inhalation, and irrigation (excluding pour bottles) in containers of 100 mL or more,
- sulfonylurea hypoglycemics, oral (e.g., chlorpropamide, glimepiride, glyburide, glipizide, tolbutamide).

Specific medications identified as high-risk are:

- epinephrine, IM, subcutaneous,
- epoprostenol (e.g., Flolan), IV,
- insulin U-500 (special emphasis*) (*All forms of insulin, subcutaneous and IV, are considered a class of high-alert medications. Insulin U-500 has been singled out for special emphasis to bring attention to the need for distinct strategies to prevent the types of errors that occur with this concentrated form of insulin),
- magnesium sulfate injection,
- methotrexate, oral, non-oncologic use,
- nitroprusside sodium for injection,
- opium tincture,
- oxytocin, IV,
- potassium chloride for injection concentrate,

- potassium phosphates injection,
- promethazine injection,
- vasopressin, IV, and intraosseous.

Another system consideration for decreasing medication errors is staff resources. Access to expert human resources on medications is needed, such as pharmacists. Medication supplies can be immediately available through unit stock or medication storage, such as electronic dispensaries. Staff need access to medication information, through either a current version of pharmacology textbooks or electronic access, such as online databases or apps. Equipment needed for medication administration should be working and accessible. Examples include IV or syringe pumps, syringes and other supplies, and bar-coded medication technology (Maryniak 2016, 2018).

Education, training, the work environment, and culture are other system considerations. Both education and experiences help to increase familiarity with commonly used medications. Didactic education for nurses is one strategy, such as inclusion in new graduate nurse residency programs. Clinical experiences include preceptorships with skilled staff to assist knowledge attainment. Work confidence through orientation to the environment can also assist. This can improve time management and decrease stress levels.

Appropriate staffing and workload are common struggles in organizations. Many organizations use ratio-based nursing, which does not consider patient acuity or level of skill of staff. Nurses who are in orientation or preceptorship should not be given full assignments until appropriate. The skill mix needs to consider licensed and unlicensed personnel. Additionally, staffing should consider how many experienced and unexperienced nurses are working during a shift.

Physical environments can impact on staff stress and well-being. These can also create distractions from the environment itself. Distractions and interruptions, as commonly identified contributors to errors, must be minimized. Some strategies include use of safe zones that are physically identified in medication rooms or around dispensaries. Other indicators to limit distractions are the use of tags to identify when a nurse is administering medications. Staff should also be empowered to safely state that he or she must focus on medication administration.

Supervision is a consideration for newer nurses, in particular, when they are learning skills around medication administration. Supportive work environments are those where nurses feel empowered and participate in shared governance. Teamwork is important to help one another learn and grow and meet the needs of patients and families. Instituting a just culture is also essential. Visible, supportive leaders who have good relationships with staff create a positive work environment. There must be trust between staff and leaders, which increases an effective culture. Fear or distrust decreases the chance that errors are effectively reported, and therefore processes are not evaluated (Maryniak 2018; Rodziewicz et al. 2021).

System considerations about the use of technology are also needed. As we grow in the use of technology in healthcare, it is important to understand that it is an additional tool to assist staff, but cannot replace critical thinking. Nurses are the last stop to safety with medication administration, and so complacency with technology can be dangerous. Bar-coded medication administration is an important strategy for medication safety. However, not all errors are caught with this technology. For example, if a nurse is to administer a partial dose, it is up to that nurse to appropriately administer the correct dose, like insulin. Additionally, the technology will not necessarily identify when a medication should not be given (such as holding a beta blocker if heart rate or blood pressure is outside parameters). Smart IV pumps are programmed with drug libraries as well as dose reduction systems (which assists with preventing inadvertent high doses). Nurse diligence can assist in identifying and verifying dosages. In one case, new IV pumps were programmed for an incorrect concentration of a medication in one facility. A nurse was verifying calculations and caught the error quickly. As a result of her diligence, all of the pumps at the facility were immediately reprogrammed with the right medication (Maryniak 2018).

Just as personal health and stress are correlated with medication errors, personal wellness is associated with better outcomes and reduced chance for errors. Staff need to ensure that they are getting adequate rest at home and taking breaks at work. It is also important not only to identify areas of stress but also to address the stress, such as the use of coping mechanisms. Staff also need to stay home from work if ill (Rodziewicz et al. 2021).

Nurses must follow the rights of medication administration each and every time. The five basic rights of medication administration are right patient, drug, time, dose, and route. Throughout the years, additional rights have been discussed, up to 12 rights in total, such as right reason, education, documentation, right to refusal, and expiration date. However, the five basic rights are consistently recommended. Nurses are also accountable for following policies and procedures. If there is unfamiliarity with policies, then referring to them should be done until familiar. Nurses should never give any medication without knowing the reason, possible side effects, interactions, safe dose range, monitoring, etc. (Rodziewicz et al. 2021).

Nurses as advocates can assist the patient and family with effective teaching, and encourage them to speak up if there are any concerns or if they do not understand something. And nurses must also listen to concerns. For example, if a patient states "Oh, the doctor said he was going to stop giving me that medication", then the nurse should verify before either administering or holding a medication. Promoting self-wellness and a supportive work culture assists everyone, including patients and families (Maryniak 2018).

Using a Daily Management System

As discussed in Chap. 5, use of a daily management system (DMS) can increase awareness, improve communication, foster transparency, help reduce errors, and improve safety. Daily management allows staff doing the work and leaders at all levels of the organization to clearly visualize whether the performance is on track (no variations) or has deviated from target condition(s). Some key points about DMS are:

- A DMS helps to rapidly identify deviation and correct the problem by bringing attention to the cause and quickly addressing the cause.
- Everyone has equal responsibility for taking necessary actions to quickly correct the problem or escalate as needed.
- Old school of thought brought attention to the problem after the fact making it difficult to find causation and fix; DMS brings immediate attention with expectation to address causation or escalate barriers as needed.

One example is focus on reducing CAUTIs. A system goal would be zero harm, with a facility goal of reducing CAUTI events. The department goal would then be decreasing the indwelling catheter days (see Fig. 6.7).

The dwell time has the highest impact on developing CAUTIs—each day increases the chance of infection. Therefore, if the dwell time can be reduced (i.e., indwelling catheter days) then CAUTIs can also be decreased.

The room number would be placed on the DMS board of patients with indwelling catheters, and these patients would be prioritized in leader rounding to ensure they meet the criteria for the catheter or it is removed. The same principle would be used for hospital-acquired pressure injuries (HAPIs) as well. Patients with a Braden score of 11 or less, for example, would be highlighted and prioritized in rounding by nurses and leaders to ensure they have adequate pressure relief interventions (see Fig. 6.8).

It is important to prioritize rounding and monitoring to aid in reduction of harm events. Whenever a patient has a device, they should be monitored closely to ensure they need the device, and if so, the processes involved with the care of the device are strictly adhered to. The only way to effectively monitor is by making this a priority. You really do get what you plan for.

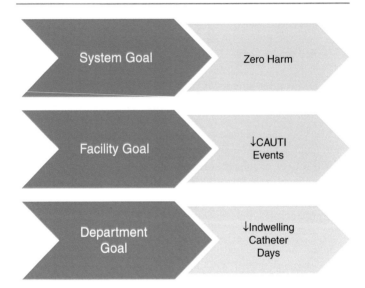

Fig. 6.7 Alignment of goals

Outcome Metric	# Since last Huddle	Days since last	Process Metric Today	Comments
Foleys > 2 days	5	NA	80%	% meets CDC criteria - target 100% Rms 320, 315, 307, 375, 310
CAUTI	1	0	80%	Bundle compliance target 90%
CLABSI	0	275	100%	CHG bath target 90%; Rms 315, 310
Falls	0	25	100%	Fall bundle compliance target 90%; High Risk: 302, 308, 319
HAPI	2	0	75%	Bundle compliance target 95%; Braden < 11: Rms 320, 315, 350, 345, 302, 316
Hand Hygiene	NA	NA	75%	Hand Hygiene target 90%

Fig. 6.8 Example of process monitoring on DMS board

References

Agency for Healthcare Research and Quality (AHRQ). (n.d.). Nurse bedside shift report: Implementation handbook. https://www.ahrq.gov/sites/default/files/wysiwyg/professionals/systems/hospital/engagingfamilies/strategy3/Strat3_Implement_Hndbook_508.pdf

Association for Professionals in Infection Control and Epidemiology (APIC) (2015). APIC implementation guide: Guide to preventing central-line associated bloodstream infections. https://apic.org/Resource_/TinyMceFileManager/2015/APIC_CLABSI_WEB.pdf

Blazin, L. J., Sitthi-Amorn, J., Hoffman, J. M., & Burlison, J. D. (2020). Improving patient handoffs and transitions through adaptation and implementation of I-PASS across multiple handoff settings. *Pediatric Quality & Safety, 5*(4), e323.

Centers for Disease Control & Prevention. (n.d.). Sequence for putting on personal protective equipment (PPE). https://www.cdc.gov/hai/pdfs/ppe/ppe-sequence.pdf

Centers for Disease Control & Prevention. (2017). Management of multidrug-resistant organisms in healthcare settings, 2006 (updated 2017). https://www.cdc.gov/infectioncontrol/pdf/guidelines/mdro-guidelines.pdf

Centers for Disease Control & Prevention. (2019). 2007 guideline for isolation precautions: Preventing transmission of infectious agents in healthcare settings (updated 2019). https://www.cdc.gov/infectioncontrol/pdf/guidelines/isolation-guidelines-H.pdf

Centers for Disease Control & Prevention. (2020). Proper N95 respirator use for respiratory protection preparedness. https://blogs.cdc.gov/niosh-science-blog/2020/03/16/n95-preparedness/

Centers for Medicare & Medicaid Services (CMS). (2020). *State operations manual: Appendix A: Survey protocol, regulations and interpretive guidelines for hospitals.* https://www.cms.gov/Regulations-and-Guidance/Guidance/Manuals/Downloads/som107ap_a_hospitals.pdf

Dorvil B. (2018). The secrets to successful nurse bedside shift report implementation and sustainability. *Nursing Management, 49*(6), 20–25.

Haesler, E. (Ed.). (2019). *Prevention and treatment of pressure ulcers/injuries: The international guideline 2019.* Cambridge Media.

Ihediohanma, B. (2020). Purposeful rounding and improved patient care: An evaluation of nurses' and nursing assistants' perceptions of purposeful rounding and intervention to improve practice. https://sigma.nursingrepository.org/bitstream/handle/10755/20948/DNPCapstone.pdf?sequence=1&isAllowed=y

Institute for Safe Medication Practices. (2018). High alert medications in acute care settings. https://www.ismp.org/recommendations/high-alert-medications-acute-list

Institute for Safe Medication Practices. (2021). ISMP's list of error-prone abbreviations, symbols, and dose designations. https://www.ismp.org/Tools/errorproneabbreviations.pdf

Jeong, I.C., Healy, R., Bao, B., Xie, W., Madeira, T., … Searson, P. (2020). Assessment of patient ambulation profiles to predict hospital readmission, discharge location, and length of stay in a cardiac surgery progressive care unit. *JAMA Network Open, 3*(3), e201074.

Klompas, M. (2019). Ventilator-associated events: What they are, and what they are not. *Respiratory Care, 64*(8), 953-961.

Krein, S. L., Mayer, J., Harrod, M., Weston, L. E., Gregory, L., Petersen, L., Samore, M. H., & Drews, F. A. (2018). Identification and characterization of failures in infectious agent transmission precaution practices in hospitals: A qualitative study. *JAMA Internal Medicine, 178*(8), 1016–1057.

LeLaurin, J., & Shorr, R. (2019). Preventing falls in hospitals: State of the science. *Clinics in Geriatric Medicine, 35*(2), 273–283.

Maryniak, K. (2016). How to avoid medication errors in nursing. https://www.rn.com/nursing-news/nurses-role-in-medication-error-prevention/

Maryniak, K. (2018). *Medication errors: Best practices for prevention* (webinar). Lorman.

Maryniak, K. (2019). *Professional nursing practice in the United States: An overview for international nurses, and those along the continuum from new graduates to experienced nurses.* Author.

Maryniak, K. (2021). *Documentation for nurses* (4th ed.) (ebook). Elite Healthcare.

Rodziewicz, T. L., Houseman, B., & Hipskind, J. E. (2021). Medical error reduction and prevention. In StatPearls. StatPearls Publishing. https://pubmed.ncbi.nlm.nih.gov/29763131/

Saint, S., Greene, T., Krein, S., Rogers, M., Ratz, D., … Gould, C. (2016). A program to prevent catheter-associated urinary tract infections in acute care. *New England Journal of Medicine, 374*, 2111-2119.

The Joint Commission. (2021a). Facts about the official "Do Not Use" list of abbreviations. https://www.jointcommission.org/facts_about_do_not_use_list/

The Joint Commission. (2021b). 2022 hospital national patient safety goals. https://www.jointcommission.org/standards/national-patient-safety-goals/hospital-national-patient-safety-goals/

Case Studies

7

Case Study #1

In a medical unit, Mr. M., a 78-year-old male, was admitted for acute COPD exacerbation. On admission, the nurse noted that Mr. M. had redness in both eyes. When asked, Mr. M. stated that he thought the eye redness was a result of seasonal allergies, as his eyes were also itchy.

Two days after Mr. M.'s admission, the patient in the next room, Mrs. W., began to have itchy, watery, red eyes. Mrs. W. was a 56-year-old female, admitted with intractable nausea and vomiting, rule out intestinal obstruction and biliary carcinoma.

The same day that Mrs. W. began with symptoms, another patient, Miss D., down the hall from Mr. M. developed these same symptoms. Miss D. was admitted for diabetic ketoacidosis and had been transferred to the medical unit from the intensive care unit two days earlier.

The charge nurse identified the trend with the patients' signs and symptoms, and called the infection preventionist. All three patients were placed in contact plus standard precautions.

The provider took cultures from the three patients, which were negative for bacteria. Acute viral conjunctivitis caused by adenovirus was confirmed for these patients through polymerase chain

K. Maryniak, R. Garrett, *Preventing Errors and Pitfalls in Nursing with Infectious Patients*, https://doi.org/10.1007/978-3-030-86728-7_7

reaction (PCR) testing, and precautions were continued throughout their hospital stays.

The nursing manager, risk manager, and infection preventionist determined that a root cause analysis would be warranted in this situation. They invited nurses, nursing assistants, a provider, and a respiratory therapist to the RCA.

- In the case of Mr. M., was there any attribution as to not recognizing he had conjunctivitis?

In this situation, signs and symptoms of acute viral conjunctivitis are itchy, watery eyes, redness, discharge, and sensitivity to light. Mr. M. stated he had seasonal allergies, which have similar symptoms. There was no attribution or wrong-doing in the missed diagnosis of conjunctivitis.

- In reviewing the spread of conjunctivitis among the medical patients, why could this happen?

The group participating in the RCA, using the five whys (Fig. 7.1), determined the contributing factors involved.

The RCA group discussed that there were appropriate processes in place, through policies and procedures, about hand

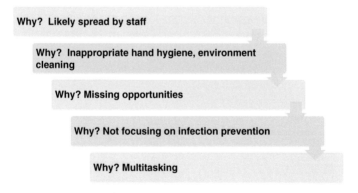

Fig. 7.1 Example of the "five whys"

hygiene and environmental cleaning. They also identified that there were appropriate equipment and supplies available for hand hygiene and environmental cleaning. Participating in the RCA, using the five whys, determined the contributing factors involved. The staff determined that the most likely cause of the cases of conjunctivitis was spread through staff. This finding aligns with statements from the CDC, that outbreaks often occur from a failure to uphold infection prevention and control practices (CDC 2021). The group admitted that there were missed opportunities for both hand hygiene and environmental cleaning among staff, including themselves. Examples included not changing gloves and performing hand hygiene when working from dirty to clean, not always performing hand hygiene at each opportunity, and not cleaning the environment (such as counters or bedside tables) at every opportunity. These behaviors were identified as at-risk, using a just culture process. Contributing factors (Table 7.1) also included the need to reinforce infection prevention practices, hold staff accountable to these practices, and communicate results from infection prevention audits.

Findings from the RCA were shared with leadership, and a corrective action plan (Table 7.2) was created to be implemented facility-wide.

Table 7.1 Contributing factors

Category	Contributing factors
People	Missing opportunities for hand hygiene and environmental cleaning; not focusing
Processes	Processes for hand hygiene and cleaning were in place
Equipment, supplies	Equipment and supplies were available
Culture	Need reinforcement of accountability for hand hygiene, appropriate use of PPE, environmental cleaning
Communication	Communication of hand hygiene audits were not done with staff
Staffing, training	Need to reinforce hand hygiene, PPE, and environmental cleaning practices

Table 7.2 Corrective action plan

Corrective action	Measure of success	Responsible party	Due to review
Reeducate staff on infection prevention measures, including reinforcing appropriate hand hygiene, use of PPE, and environmental cleaning practices	Staff will successfully pass posttest with a minimum of 80%	Clinical Education	1 month
Hand hygiene audits will be performed and results shared with staff	Audits will show 95% compliance with hand hygiene 100% of results will be posted on DMS board and reviewed with all staff	Infection Prevention	Monthly
Managers will reinforce accountability for infection prevention practices, including hand hygiene, appropriate use of PPE, environmental cleaning with staff	Infection prevention practices will be documented in staff performance reviews Progressive discipline, if warranted based on just culture, will occur for not following infection prevention practices	Managers	Ongoing

Case Study #2

A nurse leader, Jane, was rounding on the unit, and saw a new nursing assistant, Tammi, (who was just off orientation), down the hall, coming out of a patient's room. The patient was admitted for COVID 19 and was placed in droplet plus contact precautions. Tammi had full PPE on as she left the room, and began taking the PPE off outside the room. Tammi began doffing by taking off her mask, then her goggles, gown, and gloves.

When Jane reached the assistant, she asked to speak with her privately. Jane asked Tammi what education she had been given for donning and doffing PPE. Tammi stated she had only been in full

PPE once, and tried to follow what her preceptor was doing. Jane identified that this was human error and that Tammi needed more education. Jane spoke with Tammi about the importance of following the proper sequence for PPE donning and doffing, to avoid exposing herself and others to COVID 19 (CDC n.d.). Jane also realized that Tammi's preceptor might need more information.

Jane spoke with the nursing assistant preceptor, Gary. Jane learned that Gary had very little experience with donning and doffing PPE, since he had just transferred from an ambulatory setting to the medical unit with COVID patients. Gary identified that orientation felt rushed, and there were learning opportunities.

Jane worked with her educator, and they compiled an orientation guide for nursing assistants. Additionally, a competency was developed for hand hygiene, donning, and doffing PPE, for nurses and nursing assistants alike. Monthly audits were instituted following education, which showed an increase in compliance with hand hygiene and PPE.

Case Study #3

A patient, Mrs. D., was a 28-year-old female admitted to the intensive care unit with acute respiratory distress related to asthma exacerbation. She had a history of type II diabetes. Mrs. D. was never ventilated but was on high-flow nasal cannula, nebulizers, and corticosteroids. Her blood glucose levels were being monitored closely, as she was experiencing hyperglycemia. The provider ordered an indwelling urinary catheter for "strict intake and output," which was placed in the emergency room prior to the admission to ICU.

On day three, Mrs. D. was downgraded to intermediate care. However, she was kept in the ICU because there were no beds available in the IMCU. On day four, it was noted that Mrs. D.'s urine was cloudy in the collection bag, and she was complaining of pain and the need to urinate. A sterile urine sample was taken and sent to the laboratory for culture, and the indwelling catheter was removed. A diagnosis of CAUTI was confirmed. This was the fourth CAUTI in the ICU within a 3-month period of time.

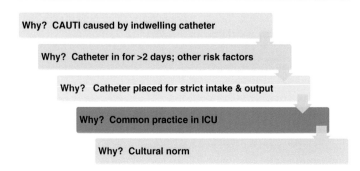

Fig. 7.2 Other example of Five whys

Although a formal RCA was not conducted, the nursing manager, infection preventionist, and risk manager did ask a group of nurses and providers to meet and discuss the case. In discussion, the group identified that the indwelling catheter was in place for more than 2 days and that the patient had other risk factors for developing an infection. They used the five whys (Fig. 7.2):

The group determined that it was a cultural norm to insert an indwelling urinary catheter in all critically ill patients for "strict intake and output." It was noted that these measurements were not needed in every patient, and the providers admitted sometimes they did not look at intake and output if it was not critical. The providers and nurses understood that CAUTIs are the most common hospital-acquired infection (Saran et al. 2018). They identified that this was at-risk behavior as a group, and was placing patients at unnecessary risk for developing CAUTIs.

The nursing and medical staff compiled a list of criteria for when an indwelling urinary catheter was critical, such as shock and trauma. They also discussed the use of external male and female urinary catheters as options for indwelling catheters. Additionally, the group determined that indwelling urinary catheter bundle compliance should be focused on. Discussion of indwelling catheters was added to the daily huddle and rounding, to keep the issue of usage at the forefront of the team members' minds.

The goals set included 90% compliance with the bundle, 100% of indwelling urinary catheters would be discussed at huddle and rounds, and 50% decrease in the use of indwelling urinary catheters over 2 days. Audits were done monthly, and after 3 months the unit met their goals. They continued to meet their goals for the remainder of the year. Additionally, the CAUTI rates decreased.

References

Centers for Disease Control & Prevention. (n.d.). Sequence for putting on personal protective equipment (PPE). https://www.cdc.gov/hai/pdfs/ppe/ppe-sequence.pdf

Centers for Disease Control and Prevention (CDC). (2021). Outbreak investigations in healthcare settings. https://www.cdc.gov/hai/outbreaks/index.html

Saran, S., Rao, N. S., & Azim, A. (2018). Diagnosing catheter-associated urinary tract infection in critically ill patients: Do the guidelines help? *Indian Journal of Critical Care Medicine, 22*(5), 357–360.

Recommendations for Further Study and Summary

8

It has been noted that there are studies that examine various errors in nursing and in healthcare. The frequency of errors directly related to infectious patients is not commonly seen in the literature. For example, there are many studies which describe hand hygiene compliance, and some regarding compliance with personal protective equipment. There are gaps in the literature regarding the correlation between noncompliance or errors with hand hygiene and PPE, and rates of hospital outbreaks, staff illness, or other contagious effects.

Additionally, studies have been done regarding errors that contribute to falls, hospital-acquired conditions, and medication errors. There is an opportunity to examine the frequency of these types of errors in combination with patients in isolation or on precautions. There are more requirements in caring for acutely ill infectious patients, which may lead to more contributing factors that can lead to errors. The work environment, stress, additional time constraints, and current changes in the workforce can increase the risk of errors with infectious patients. There may also be additional stacking in the minds of nurses caring for these patients, which can also lead to errors.

There are also opportunities to further delve into specific system and personal contributing factors and errors that occur.

© The Author(s), under exclusive license to Springer Nature Switzerland AG 2022
K. Maryniak, R. Garrett, *Preventing Errors and Pitfalls in Nursing with Infectious Patients*, https://doi.org/10.1007/978-3-030-86728-7_8

Examining organizational traits, including staffing practices, use of skill mix, and incorporation of best practices into policies and procedures compared with error rates can provide valuable information. Looking at personal considerations, including years of experience, education, certification, and leader qualities correlating with rates of errors are also needed.

Examining personal effects of errors from the perspective of the infectious patient, family, and nurse is also required. Both quantitative and qualitative studies would add significance to this topic.

Summary

Caring for patients with infectious diseases requires complex nursing care. Baseline knowledge about common infections is essential for nursing staff. There are errors that can occur directly related to the infectious processes, such as inappropriate or omitted hand hygiene, or the donning and doffing of personal protective equipment. Infectious patients are also at risk for other nursing errors, such as medication errors, falls, or hospital-acquired conditions.

There are multiple factors that can contribute to nursing errors, both at system and personal levels. Organizations, leaders, and staff together are accountable for ensuring there are appropriate processes for reducing the risk of errors. Diligence, communication, and a constant focus on safety are required.

Potential or actual errors can create a near-miss situation or one with actual harm. The consequences of nursing errors can be detrimental to many people, not just the patient. Patients, families, and healthcare professionals can all be affected by errors.

Effective systems must be in place to properly monitor for and detect nursing errors. These systems should be beneficial to all key stakeholders, and add value to processes. Use of a just culture in an organization is also needed for reporting, monitoring, and creating change.

Nurses should also keep up to date with evidence-based practices. The use of bundles, strategies for alternatives to invasive procedures, and purposeful rounding are all examples. As health-care continues to evolve and research is done, changes in practice will continue to focus on what is learned to provide the best qual-ity care to patients.

References

Adler, L., Yi, D., Li, M., McBroom, B., Hauck, L., ... & Classen, D. (2018). Impact of inpatient harms on hospital finances and patient clinical outcomes. *Journal of Patient Safety, 14*(2), 67-73

Afreen, N., Padilla-Tolentino, E., & McGinnis, B. (2021). Identifying potential high-risk medication errors using telepharmacy and a web-based survey tool. *Innovations in Pharmacy, 12*(1), 10.

Agency for Healthcare Research & Quality. (2018). Never events. https://psnet.ahrq.gov/primers/primer/3/never-events%5D%20since

Al-ghraiybah, T., Sim, J., & Lago, L. (2021). The relationship between the nursing practice environment and five nursing-sensitive patient outcomes in acute care hospitals: A systematic review. *Nursing Open, 8*(5), 2262-2271.

American Society for Healthcare Risk Management. (2014). Serious safety events: A focus on harm classification: Deviation in care as link. http://www.ashrm.org/pubs/files/white_papers/SSE-2_getting_to_zero-9-30-14.pdf

Asia Pacific Society of Infection Control. (2015). APSIC guide for prevention of central line associated bloodstream infections (CLABSI). https://apsic-apac.org/wp-content/uploads/2016/09/APSIC-CLABSI-guidelines-FINAL-20-Jan-2015.pdf

Association for Professionals in Infection Control and Epidemiology (APIC) (2015). APIC implementation guide: Guide to preventing central-line associated bloodstream infections. https://apic.org/Resource_/TinyMce-FileManager/2015/APIC_CLABSI_WEB.pdf

Ayoade, F. (2021). Herpes simplex. https://emedicine.medscape.com/article/218580-overview

Bigani, D. K., & Correia, A. M. (2018). On the same page: Nurse, patient, and family perceptions of change-of-shift bedside report. *Journal of Pediatric Nursing, 41*, 84–89.

K. Maryniak, R. Garrett, *Preventing Errors and Pitfalls in Nursing with Infectious Patients*, https://doi.org/10.1007/978-3-030-86728-7

Blazin, L. J., Sitthi-Amorn, J., Hoffman, J. M., & Burlison, J. D. (2020). Improving patient handoffs and transitions through adaptation and implementation of I-PASS across multiple handoff settings. *Pediatric Quality & Safety, 5(*4), e323.

Bocka, J. (2019). Pertussis. https://emedicine.medscape.com/article/967268-overview

Brown, N., Reacher, M., Rice, W., Roddick, I., Reeve, L., … & Enoch, D. (2019). An outbreak of methicillin-resistant staphylococcus aureus colonization in a neonatal intensive care unit: use of a case-control study to investigate and control it and lessons learnt. *Journal of Hospital Infections, 103*(1), 35-43.

Buensalido, J. (2019). Rhinovirus (RV) infection (common cold). https://emedicine.medscape.com/article/227820-overview

Bush, M., & Vazquez-Pertejo, M. (2021). Staphylococcal infections. Merck Manual. https://www.merckmanuals.com/professional/infectious-diseases/gram-positive-cocci/staphylococcal-infections

Cennimo, D. (2019). Parvovirus B19 infection. https://emedicine.medscape.com/article/961063-overview

Centers for Disease Control & Prevention. (n.d.). Sequence for putting on personal protective equipment (PPE). https://www.cdc.gov/hai/pdfs/ppe/ppe-sequence.pdf

Centers for Disease Control & Prevention. (2017). Management of multidrug-resistant organisms in healthcare settings, 2006 (updated 2017). https://www.cdc.gov/infectioncontrol/pdf/guidelines/mdro-guidelines.pdf

Centers for Disease Control & Prevention. (2019). 2007 guideline for isolation precautions: Preventing transmission of infectious agents in healthcare settings (updated 2019). https://www.cdc.gov/infectioncontrol/pdf/guidelines/isolation-guidelines-H.pdf

Centers for Disease Control & Prevention. (2021a). About COVID 19. https://www.cdc.gov/coronavirus/2019-ncov/your-health/about-covid-19.html

Centers for Disease Control & Prevention. (2021b). Chickenpox (varicella) for healthcare professionals. https://www.cdc.gov/chickenpox/hcp/index.html

Centers for Disease Control and Prevention (CDC). (2021). Outbreak investigations in healthcare settings. https://www.cdc.gov/hai/outbreaks/index.html

Centers for Medicare & Medicaid Services (CMS). (2020). *State operations manual: Appendix A: Survey protocol, regulations and interpretive guidelines for hospitals.* https://www.cms.gov/Regulations-and-Guidance/Guidance/Manuals/Downloads/som107ap_a_hospitals.pdf

Centers for Medicare & Medicaid Services (CMS). (2021). *Specifications manual, version 5.11a: Discharges 01/01/2022 to 06/30/2022.* https://qualitynet.cms.gov/inpatient/specifications-manuals

Chen, S. (2019). Measles. https://emedicine.medscape.com/article/966220-overview#a5

Davis, T., DeWalt, D., Hink, A., Hawk, V., Brega, A., & Mabachi, N. (2020). Health literacy: Hidden barriers and practical strategies. https://www.ahrq.gov/professionals/quality-patient-safety/quality-resources/tools/literacy-toolkit/tool3a/index.html

Defendi, G. (2019). Mumps. https://reference.medscape.com/article/966678-overview

Donaldson L., Ricciardi W., Sheridan, S., & Tartaglia, R. (eds). (2021). *Textbook of patient safety and clinical risk management*. Springer.

Dorvil B. (2018). The secrets to successful nurse bedside shift report implementation and sustainability. *Nursing Management, 49*(6), 20–25.

Ezike, E. (2017). Pediatric rubella clinical presentation. https://emedicine.medscape.com/article/968523-clinical

Fan, J., Jiang, Y., Hu, K., Chen, X., Xu, Q., … & Liang, S. (2020). Barriers to using personal protective equipment by healthcare staff during the COVID-19 outbreak in China. *Medicine, 99*(48), e23310.

Godshall, M. (2018). Preventing medication errors in the information age. *Nursing, 48*(9), 56-58.

Grinspan, A. (2021). C. difficile infection. American College of Gastroenterology. https://gi.org/topics/c-difficile-infection/

Guenther, L. (2019). Pediculosis and pthiriasis (lice infestation). https://emedicine.medscape.com/article/225013-overview

Haesler, E. (Ed.). (2019). *Prevention and treatment of pressure ulcers/injuries: The international guideline 2019*. Cambridge Media.

He, Q., Wang, W., Zhu, S., Wang, M., Kang, Y., … & Sun, X. (2021). The epidemiology and clinical outcomes of ventilator-associated events among 20,769 mechanically ventilated patients at intensive care units: An observational study. *Critical Care, 25*(44). https://ccforum.biomedcentral.com/articles/10.1186/s13054-021-03484-x#citeas

Henriques, V. (2018). Medication management. The Joint Commission. https://www.jointcommission.org/assets/1/6/Medication_Management_Presentation.pdf

Herchline, T. (2020). Tuberculosis (TB). https://emedicine.medscape.com/article/230802-overview

Huang, H., Ran, J., Yang, J., Li, P., Zhuang, G. (2019). Impact of MRSA transmission and infection in a neonatal intensive care unit in China: A bundle intervention study during 2014-2017. *BioMed Research International*, 2019. https://www.hindawi.com/journals/bmri/2019/5490413/

Ihediohanma, B. (2020). Purposeful rounding and improved patient care: An evaluation of nurses' and nursing assistants' perceptions of purposeful rounding and intervention to improve practice. https://sigma.nursingrepository.org/bitstream/handle/10755/20948/DNPCapstone.pdf?sequence=1&isAllowed=y

Institute for Safe Medication Practices. (2018). High alert medications in acute care settings. https://www.ismp.org/recommendations/high-alert-medications-acute-list

Institute for Safe Medication Practices. (2021). ISMP's list of error-prone abbreviations, symbols, and dose designations. https://www.ismp.org/Tools/errorproneabbreviations.pdf

Institute of Medicine. (2000). *To err is human: Building a safer health system*. National Academies Press.

International Society on Thrombosis and Haemostasis. (2022). Open your eyes to venous thromboembolism (VTE). https://www.worldthrombosis-day.org/issue/vte/

Janniger, C. (2021). Herpes zoster. https://emedicine.medscape.com/article/1132465-overview

Jeong, I.C., Healy, R., Bao, B., Xie, W., Madeira, T., … & Searson, P. (2020). Assessment of patient ambulation profiles to predict hospital readmission, discharge location, and length of stay in a cardiac surgery progressive care unit. *JAMA Network Open, 3*(3), e201074.

Johns Hopkins Medicine. (2016). Study suggests medical errors now third leading cause of death in the U.S. https://www.hopkinsmedicine.org/news/media/releases/study_suggests_medical_errors_now_third_leading_cause_of_death_in_the_us

Khan, Z. (2018). Norovirus. https://emedicine.medscape.com/article/224225-overview

Khan, Z. (2021). Group A streptococcus (GAS) infections. https://emedicine.medscape.com/article/228936-overview

Klompas, M. (2019). Ventilator-associated events: What they are, and what they are not. *Respiratory Care, 64*(8), 953-961.

Krein, S. L., Mayer, J., Harrod, M., Weston, L. E., Gregory, L., Petersen, L., Samore, M. H., & Drews, F. A. (2018). Identification and characterization of failures in infectious agent transmission precaution practices in hospitals: A qualitative study. *JAMA Internal Medicine, 178*(8), 1016–1057.

Krilov, L. (2019). Respiratory syncytial virus infection. https://emedicine.medscape.com/article/971488-overview

Lanzieri, T., Redd, S., Abernathy, E., & Icenogle, J. (2020). *Manual for the surveillance of vaccine-preventable diseases: Chapter 15: Congenital rubella syndrome*. https://www.cdc.gov/vaccines/pubs/surv-manual/chpt15-crs.html

Lee, T.-K., Välimäki, M., & Lantta, T. (2021). The knowledge, practice and attitudes of nurses regarding physical restraint: Survey results from psychiatric inpatient settings. *International Journal of Environmental Research and Public Health, 18*(13).

LeLaurin, J., & Shorr, R. (2019). Preventing falls in hospitals: State of the science. *Clinics in Geriatric Medicine, 35*(2), 273–283.

Letica-Kriegel, A. S., Salmasian, H., Vawdrey, D. K., Youngerman, B. E., Green, R. A., Furuya, E. Y., Calfee, D. P., & Perotte, R. (2019). Identifying the risk factors for catheter-associated urinary tract infections: a large cross-sectional study of six hospitals. *BMJ Open, 9*(2), e022137.

Li, Z, Lina, F., Thalibb, L, & Chaboyera, W. (2020). Global prevalence and incidence of pressure injuries in hospitalised adult patients: A systematic review and meta-analysis. *International Journal of Nursing Studies, 105*. https://www.sciencedirect.com/science/article/pii/S0020748920300316?via%3Dihub

Lo, B. (2019). Diphtheria. https://emedicine.medscape.com/article/782051-overview

MacDowell, P., Cabri, A., & Davis, M. (2021). Medication administration errors. Patient Safety Network. https://psnet.ahrq.gov/primer/medication-administration-errors

Makini, S., Umschied, C., Soo, J., Chu, V., Barlett, A., Landon, E., & Marrs, R. (2021). Hand hygiene compliance rate during the COVID-19 pandemic. *JAMA Internal Medicine, 181*(7), 1006-1008.

Marx, D. (2001). *Patient safety and the just culture: A primer for health care executives.* Trustees of Columbia University.

Maryniak, K. (2016). How to avoid medication errors in nursing. https://www.rn.com/nursing-news/nurses-role-in-medication-error-prevention/

Maryniak, K. (2018). *Medication errors: Best practices for prevention* (webinar). Lorman.

Maryniak, K. (2019). *Professional nursing practice in the United States: An overview for international nurses, and those along the continuum from new graduates to experienced nurses.* Author.

Maryniak, K. (2021). *Documentation for nurses* (4th ed.) (ebook). Elite Healthcare.

Miller, D. (2021). I-PASS as a nursing communication tool. *Pediatric Nursing, 47*(1), 30–37.

National Institutes of Health. (2021). COVID-19 treatment guidelines. https://www.covid19treatmentguidelines.nih.gov

Nguyen, D. (2018). Rotavirus. https://emedicine.medscape.com/article/803885-overview#a4

Nicastri, E., & Leone, S. (2021). Guide to infection control in the healthcare setting: Healthcare associated urinary tract infections. https://isid.org/guide/hospital/urinary-tract-infections/

Office of Disease Prevention and Health Promotion. (2018). Overview: Adverse drug events. https://health.gov/hcq/ade.asp

Ozeke, O., Ozeke, V., Coskun, O., & Budakoglu, I. I. (2019). Second victims in health care: current perspectives. *Advances in Medical Education and Practice, 10*, 593–603.

Öztürk R, Murt A. (2020). Epidemiology of urological infections: A global burden. *World Journal of Urology, 38*(11), 2669-2679.

Panagioti, M., Khan, K., Keers, R., Abuzour, A., Phipps, D., … & Ashcroft, D. (2019). Prevalence, severity, and nature of preventable patient harm across medical care settings: Systematic review and meta-analysis. *BMJ, 366,* l4185.

Papadakis, M.A., McPhee, S.J., & Bernstein, J. (Eds.), (2020). *Quick medical diagnosis & treatment 2020*. McGraw Hill.

Papadopoulos, A. (2020). Chickenpox. https://emedicine.medscape.com/article/1131785-overview

Paradiso, L., & Sweeney, N. (2019). Just culture. *Nursing Management 50*(6), 38-45.

Popoola, V., Budd, A., Wittig, S., Ross, T., Aucott, S., ... & Milstone, A. M. (2014). Methicillin-resistant staphylococcus aureus transmission and infections in a neonatal intensive care unit despite active surveillance cultures and decolonization: Challenges for infection prevention. *Infection Control and Hospital Epidemiology, 35*(4), 412–418.

PSNet. (2019). Medication errors and adverse drug events. https://psnet.ahrq.gov/primer/medication-errors-and-adverse-drug-events

Rodziewicz, T. L., Houseman, B., & Hipskind, J. E. (2021). Medical error reduction and prevention. In StatPearls. StatPearls Publishing. https://pubmed.ncbi.nlm.nih.gov/29763131/

Rogers, E., Griffin, E., Carnie, W., Melucci, J., & Weber, R. J. (2017). A Just culture approach to managing medication errors. *Hospital Pharmacy, 52*(4), 308–315.

Roth, C., Brewer, M., & Wieck, K. L. (2017). Using a Delphi method to identify human factors contributing to nursing errors. *Nursing Forum, 52*(3), 173–179.

Saint, S., Greene, T., Krein, S., Rogers, M., Ratz, D., ... Gould C (2016). A program to prevent catheter-associated urinary tract infections in acute care. *New England Journal of Medicine, 374*, 2111-2119.

Salar, A., Kiani, F., & Rezaee, N. (2020). Preventing the medication errors in hospitals: A qualitative study. *International Journal of Africa Nursing Sciences, 13.*

Samji, N. (2017). Viral hepatitis. https://emedicine.medscape.com/article/775507-overview

Saran, S., Rao, N. S., & Azim, A. (2018). Diagnosing catheter-associated urinary tract infection in critically ill patients: Do the guidelines help? *Indian Journal of Critical Care Medicine, 22*(5), 357–360.

Scott, I. (2020). Viral conjunctivitis (pink eye). https://emedicine.medscape.com/article/1191370-overview

Smith, C. (2017). First, do no harm: Institutional betrayal and trust in health care organizations. *Journal of Multidisciplinary Healthcare, 10*, 133-144.

Stephenson, M., Mcarthur, A., Giles, K., Lockwood, C., Aromataris, E., & Pearson, A. (2016). Prevention of falls in acute hospital settings: A multisite audit and best practice implementation project. *International Journal for Quality in Health Care, 28*(1), 92–98.

Sweeney, B. (2016). *Lean six sigma quickstart guide: The simplified beginner's guide to lean six sigma*. ClydeBank Media.

Taylor, T.A., & Unakal, C.G. (2021). Staphylococcus aureus. In: StatPearls https://www.ncbi.nlm.nih.gov/books/NBK441868/

The College of Physicians of Philadelphia. (2019). Rubella. https://www.historyofvaccines.org/content/articles/rubella

The Joint Commission. (2021a). Facts about the official "Do Not Use" list of abbreviations. https://www.jointcommission.org/facts_about_do_not_use_list/

The Joint Commission. (2021b). 2022 hospital national patient safety goals. https://www.jointcommission.org/standards/national-patient-safety-goals/hospital-national-patient-safety-goals/

Thomas, L., Donohue-Porter, P., & Fishbein, J. (2017). Impact of interruptions, distractions, and cognitive load on procedure failures and medication administration errors. *Journal of Nursing Care Quality, 32*(4), 309-317.

U.S. Department of Health and Human Services. (2021). Catheter-associated urinary tract infections. https://arpsp.cdc.gov/profile/infections/cauti?redirect=true

U.S. Food & Drug Administration. (2019). Working to reduce medication errors. https://www.fda.gov/drugs/resourcesforyou/consumers/ucm143553.htm

U.S. Food & Drug Administration. (2021). Medication errors related to CDER-regulated drug products. https://www.fda.gov/Drugs/DrugSafety/MedicationErrors/default.htm

Vasudeva, S. (2021). Meningitis. https://emedicine.medscape.com/article/232915-overview

Walsh, C., Liang, L., Grogan, T., Coles, C., McNair, N., & Nuckols, T. (2018). Temporal trends in fall rates with the implementation of a multifaceted fall prevention program: Persistence pays off. *The Joint Commission Journal on Quality and Patient Safety, 44*(1), 75-83.